Balancing

Breast & Bottle:

Reaching Your Breastfeeding Goals

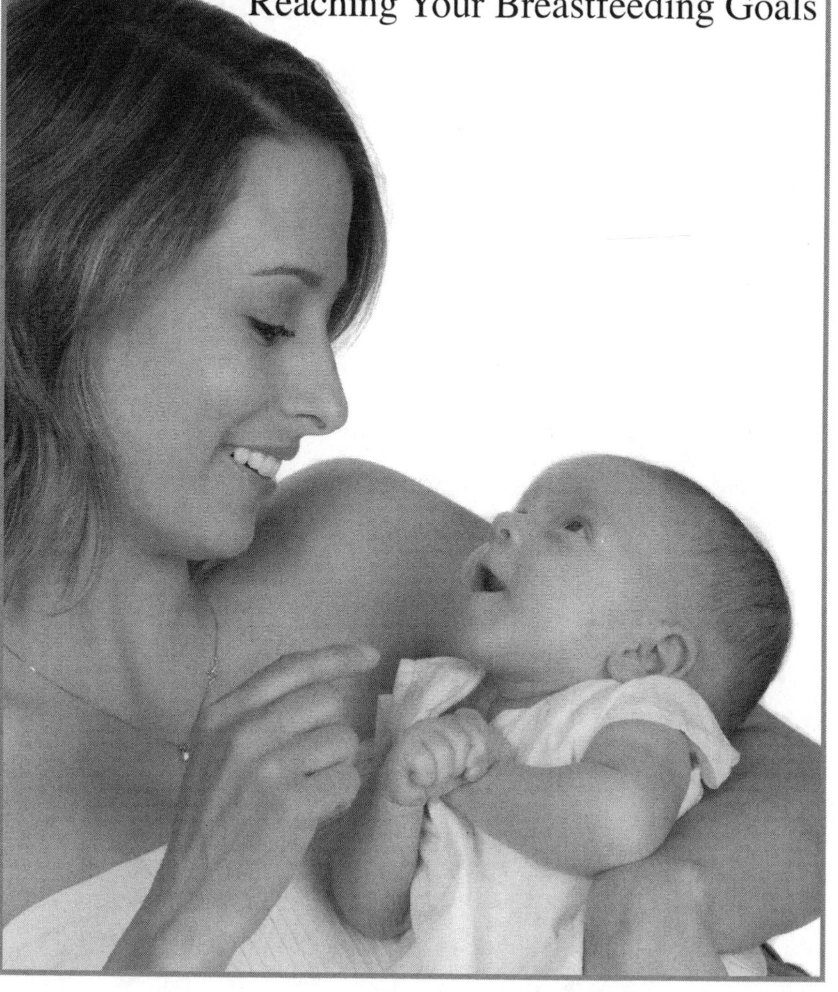

Balancing Breast and Bottle:

Reaching Your Breastfeeding Goals

Amy Peterson, BS, IBCLC
Mindy Harmer, MA, CCC-SLP

Hale Publishing
1825 E Plano Parkway, Suite 280
Plano, TX 75074

Balancing Breast and Bottle:
Reaching Your Breastfeeding Goals

Amy Peterson, BS, IBCLC
Mindy Harmer, MA, CCC-SLP

Hale Publishing, L.P.
1825 E. Plano Parkway, Suite 280
Plano, TX 7950741
978-578-0400
800-378-1317
www.HalePublishing.com

Library of Congress Control Number: 2009939406
ISBN-13: 978-0-9823379-5-0

Printed by Edwards Brothers Malloy

Table of Contents

Acknowledgements

We gratefully acknowledge the many people who influenced our writing. We would like to express our deepest gratitude to the mothers who shared their stories and their sweet babies. Thank you, Baby Caroline who refused to take a bottle, and Baby Kayla who refused to take the breast; many other babies will be successful because of your mothers' patience and persistence. Cathy Watson Genna, thank you for spending time talking shop and your thoughtful suggestions. Diana West and Lisa Marasco, we appreciate you sharing an early peek at your fabulous book. Lisa Sandora and Karen Gromada, thanks for sharing your bottle nipple study with us; this helped us form the direction of our bottle-nipple-flow study without reinventing the wheel. Thank you, Anita Bartels, for your help accessing research. Kathy Kendall-Tackett, thank you so much for taking interest in our ideas and inviting a second look. Janet Rourke and the rest of our support team at Hale Publishing, thank you for patiently introducing us to the publishing process.

Amy's Personal Acknowledgements

Linda Smith, my first mentor, thank you for suggesting all the right people to launch this project. Summer Stout-Bloyer, whom I admire in every way, thanks for being my personal cheerleader. My friend Cathy Watson-Genna, I appreciate sharing ideas with you and look forward to many more conversations. Thank you, Mindy, for getting on my train; our combined knowledge and technique never ceases to amaze me. I am thankful for La Leche League, which provided me with the tools to lay my foundation of mothering and invaluable communication skills. Thanks to my family... mom and dad, Kathy and Bob Welty, for listening to and supporting this seemingly endless, consuming project. Love to my precious children, Amanda, Ryan, Cody, and Steven—my life has changed in the best way because of you; thanks for patiently waiting for my attention during the writing process (and for your turn on the computer!). My husband Pete, who is more knowledgeable about breastfeeding than most mothers, thank you for sharing my excitement and providing me with the privilege of staying home to be a mom, my first career choice. Highest thanks to my Savior, who teaches me daily that all things do work together for good.

Mindy's Personal Acknowledgements

I am forever thankful to my parents, Mike and Mickey Harmer, for the frequent care of their grandchildren, so I could successfully juggle career and motherhood. Thank you to my dear friend, mentor, and business partner (in that order), Cherri Suter, who always makes me laugh and has time for me to vent and problem solve. Kate Dersch, thanks for believing the book would come to fruition and for your willingness to banter ideas. Dr. Katarina Haley, my long time friend, thank you for inspiring me to do more professionally. I am thankful for my sweet son Colton, who as a baby enjoyed round the clock nursing and full bottles of breastmilk; you were the inspiration for many of the ideas covered in this book. Lacey, my darling daughter, thank you for giving up your mommy-time while I worked on this book and for all the times you asked, "How's your book going?" My husband Eric, I appreciate your love and support.

Foreword

No one could have prepared me for the emotional impact of breastfeeding my children – my pride at their growing bodies and minds (that was ALL from ME!), the way my heart leapt when my baby let go for a moment to smile at me, milk dribbling down her cheek, how quickly nursing soothed fussiness or helped lull him into sleep. If you've gotten past the challenging early learning days, you know what breastfeeding means to you and your baby.

If you are reading this book because you are expecting a baby, you likely have a glimmer that you want to continue this relationship even though you know you are going to be separated from your baby for part of the day. This book will show you how you can put your milk in a bottle for some feedings and still keep breastfeeding. If you are already having difficulties with a baby going between bottle and breast, this book can help you analyze the problem and make bottle-feeding more like breastfeeding for your baby.

Babies suck differently at the breast and from a bottle. Before this book, all that parents had to guide them were marketing claims or friends' experiences. How could radically different bottles each be the "best" for breastfeeding babies? Of course, babies are different, and the best choice for any one baby will be unique. Amy and Mindy (an International Board Certified Lactation Consultant and a Speech and Language Pathologist, respectively) have worked together for years to help solve sucking problems in babies. They understand what things are important for breastfeeding mothers to know when they need to use a bottle. They use many photos and examples to help make it easier to choose a bottle, and use the bottle in a way that supports breastfeeding. So you can keep those sweet, milky smiles coming when you are with your baby, and know that your baby is getting at least a part of you when you are separated.

Cathy Watson-Genna

Preface

If you picked up this book, chances are you are already committed to breastfeeding and find yourself in need of an alternate feeding method. In today's economic times, more and more breastfeeding mothers are finding themselves returning to the workforce. Despite separation between mother and baby, many mothers wish to continue breastfeeding. Although they can find valuable information regarding collecting and storing breastmilk in many texts and online, information on how to feed their babies breastmilk during separation remains elusive. Common suggestions found in breastfeeding books include cup or syringe feeding, neither of which is practical for multiple feedings in most child-care settings.

Our combined professions of International Board Certified Lactation Consultant and Speech Language Pathologist bring two unique perspectives in solving the dilemma of how to feed a breastfed baby during separation and continue to protect the breastfeeding relationship. We also bring the viewpoint of our experiences: Amy as a stay-at-home mother and Mindy as a mother employed outside the home. We present valuable information in concise chapters, so that a busy mom can quickly find the information she needs, leaving her more time to be with her baby.

Both Amy and Mindy have breastfed their little boy and girl babies. We love them equally, but for clarity in *Balancing Breast and Bottle*, we refer to all babies as "he" and all mothers as "she."

Introduction

Every family is different. Mothers who are near their babies throughout the day may never need to select a bottle or a pacifier. However, mothers who breastfeed their babies and are employed outside the home will usually need a second feeding and comfort method. There are also mothers who, in balancing the many demands of motherhood, choose to use a second feeding or comfort method for their babies. The most common and efficient way for others to feed your baby is with a bottle. The most common and efficient way for others to satisfy your baby's desire to suck is with a pacifier. This leaves mothers to select a bottle and a pacifier for their breastfed babies that do not undermine breastfeeding.

We surveyed numerous mothers to understand how bottle nipples were commonly chosen for their breastfed babies. We discovered that bottle selection was often based on advertising, word of mouth, or hospital samples. The purchase of a bottle system can be daunting because there are so many bottle nipple choices on the market, many claiming to be "most like breastfeeding." Some bottle nipples even look like a breast, but just because they look like a breast does not mean they function like a breast. Bottle-feeding "depends not only on the characteristics of the nipple, but also on the forces generated by the infant" (Matthew, 1988, p. 688).

It would be wonderful if there were a product on the market that could simulate breastfeeding. The truth is nothing can mimic the interaction between a mom's milk supply, her breast shape, and her baby's suck. This interaction is exclusive to each mother and baby. Every mother's breast has a unique shape, texture, and flow. Every baby has a slightly different suck. Bottle nipples need to be chosen to best fit each mother/baby pair.

The baby product market is a billion-dollar industry. Many of these baby companies give free pacifiers and bottles to hospitals. When a hospital gives these free samples to new parents, the parents may think these brands are the preferred or better-quality product. Walker (2001) states that 95% of families buy the same brand of formula that the hospital gives them. Baby product distributors rely on brand recognition and loyalty, which is why some packaging states *most trusted in hospitals*.

Current lactation books contain comprehensive chapters on pumping and storing breastmilk. There may even be a page or two within these books about how to introduce a bottle. However, these pages are almost always followed by paragraphs warning the nursing mom that bottle-feeding can be detrimental to breastfeeding. The studies supporting the relationship between bottle-feeding and early weaning have prompted an absence in the literature regarding the selection and use of bottles. This literary black hole, and sometimes misinformation, can cause much mommy stress. Nursing moms have to have a way to feed their babies while they are away. We have all heard stories about babies who have cried for hours because they were unwilling to take a bottle while in another person's care. No mother wants her baby to ever feel this upset. Breastfeeding mothers need information on how to choose and use bottles and pacifiers.

You can find this information in *Balancing Breast and Bottle*. In reading our book, you will understand the special nuances of breastfeeding your baby and learn how bottle-feeding can relate to breastfeeding. It is possible for you to learn to balance breastfeeding and bottle-feeding without sabotaging your breastfeeding goals.

There is much to be explored in finding the best way to feed and comfort your baby when the two of you are apart. In this book, you will first learn why breastmilk is best and review the basics of breastfeeding and collecting milk. Then you will learn about the qualities of your baby's suck and how to choose the best bottle nipple or pacifier for *your* baby's suck. You will study the interplay between breastfeeding and artificial nipple use, looking at the ideal balance and many other suggestions, so you can find balance for your own family. You will discover what it takes to reach your breastfeeding goal and perhaps even extend your goal. Finally, you will have the information you need to remove the worry of, "Will my baby eat when we are apart?"

As you read, learn, and discover what works best for your baby, we invite you to share your experience on our website, www.breastandbottlefeeding.com. To learn more about products mentioned in *Balancing Breast and Bottle*, visit our website.

SECTION 1

First Things First

Chapter 1
Breastmilk is Best

Learning how to maintain breastfeeding while introducing and using bottles is the heart of this book and most certainly the reason you purchased it. You might be tempted to jump right to the section that contains this valuable information. Please feel free if you have been successfully breastfeeding for three weeks and your milk supply is well established. However, if you are just beginning to explore breastfeeding or have a baby younger than three weeks old, please read Section 1 to ensure breastfeeding is going well. Balancing breast and bottle-feedings is dependent upon successful breastfeeding. We begin with the importance of using your milk—information that may encourage you to stay the course when life becomes hectic.

The American Academy of Pediatrics (AAP, 2005), the World Health Organization (WHO, 2009), and many other national health agencies agree that exclusive breastfeeding (only breastmilk) for six months is vital for optimal health outcomes. Babies younger than six months of age do not need water; breastmilk is 88% water (WHO, 2009). Even in the summer months, young babies do not need water. Recognizing that a baby might not feed at the breast for every feeding, the *Global Strategy for Infant and Young Child Feeding* (WHO, 2003) recommends food choices for babies, written here from the healthiest choice to the least healthy choice:

- Mother's own fresh milk
- Mother's thawed, previously frozen milk
- Pasteurized breastmilk from a donor mother or milk bank
- Breastmilk substitute (formula)

How fascinating that breastmilk is rated as the top three choices of baby milk. Breastmilk is often called nature's perfect food. It is species-specific. Dogs drink dog milk, horses drink horse milk, dolphins drink dolphin milk, and humans drink human milk. When a baby receives breastmilk, this is "normal" and a superior choice over using any milk substitute.

Breastmilk is best for human babies because it contains the exact nutrition and antibodies babies need to stay healthy, and it is easier to digest than formula. Breastfed babies are sick less often. Children who were breastfed are less likely to develop severe lower respiratory tract infections, atopic dermatitis, or diabetes, or to become obese (Ip et al., 2007). The long-term impact of breastfeeding includes better school performance, increased productivity, and improved intellectual and social development (WHO, 2003). The longer a baby receives his mother's milk, the healthier he will be.

Breastfeeding is also best for you, the mother. Breastfeeding your baby burns extra calories. It helps guard against postpartum depression and reduces the risk of many health problems, such as osteoporosis, anemia, and breast and ovarian cancer (Ip et al., 2007).

Not only is breastfeeding best for baby and mother, it is also best for the family and the environment. It is estimated that American families can save $1,500 per year by breastfeeding (United States Breastfeeding Committee, 2002). Breastfeeding is green—there is no energy used to produce, package, and ship products and no packaging waste with breastmilk. Everyone benefits when babies breastfeed.

Knowing the positive results that come from your efforts can feel motivating during times when breastfeeding might seem overwhelming or when well-meaning friends or critics question your hard work. Clearly, breastmilk is best.

Mothers who choose to breastfeed their babies also know there are potential risks associated with formula. The most well-known health risks associated with formula use include: an increased incidence of ear infections and diarrhea, pediatric and adult onset diabetes, and obesity. The risk of eczema, food allergies, and asthma increases when there is a family history of these ailments (United States Breastfeeding Committee, 2002).

There also are lesser-known, immediate risks from the introduction of formula. First, formula can cause babies to have an upset tummy, exhibited by crying and spitting up. Secondly, frequent formula feedings can lead to constipation in some babies, with juice being the recommended solution, but you have just read that juice should be avoided for the first 6 months. Moreover, formula use without pumping the breasts sets in motion lower milk production. These risks are worrisome.

Naturally, some mothers feel guilty or concerned if they find themselves in a position of adding formula to their baby's diet. Sadly, some mothers give up breastfeeding at this point, thinking that the benefits of breastmilk are cancelled by adding formula. But this is not true; breastfeeding need not be "all or none." Continuing to provide breastmilk, alongside occasional formula use when needed, is valuable.

Delaying the introduction of formula for as long as possible can reduce the potential risks of its use. A delay in introduction allows your baby's digestive system time to mature. To date, there are no studies that confirm how much supplementation a baby can receive without harming the natural environment of a breastfed baby's intestines. Waiting at least three weeks is beneficial; waiting six weeks is a better choice; and so on. You can reduce the risks associated with formula by providing breastmilk exclusively for as long as possible—the best choice. Continuing to provide breastmilk, alongside occasional formula use, is the next-best choice. Some breastmilk is always better than no breastmilk.

Chapter 2
How to Breastfeed in a Nutshell

Breastfeeding is the most natural way to feed your baby, though it may not come naturally. That is why there are breastfeeding classes, numerous comprehensive breastfeeding books, and great websites available to mothers. We encourage you to borrow or purchase, and read, at least one recently published comprehensive breastfeeding book in addition to this book. Appendix A contains a list of some our favorites. Despite the availability of information on how to get started breastfeeding, we feel it is important to include some of the information we find most relevant. We have selected and condensed breastfeeding basics to assist you in getting started.

In this chapter, you will learn how to arouse your baby for feedings, look for and understand baby hunger cues, and select a feeding style and position that works best for you and your baby. You will also learn positive signs that breastfeeding is going well and ways to avoid overly full breasts. Finally, because not all babies are born fabulous feeders, you may need to seek extra help. Our list of red flags will help you determine when you need assistance.

Childbirth Can Influence Breastfeeding

Attending a childbirth preparation class is beneficial. Research shows that babies are more alert for breastfeeding after an unmedicated birth (Ransjo-Arvidson et al., 2001). Taking a childbirth preparation class before your baby is born may equip you with the tools you need to avoid medication. Many babies breastfeed without complication, even when a birth includes an epidural or ends in a cesarean section. Be prepared, do the best you can, and know your baby can learn to breastfeed regardless of whether you have an ideal birth experience or not. After your baby is born, keeping your baby in close proximity (rooming-in) in the hospital, rather than going back and forth to the nursery, will support breastfeeding.

Waking the Baby for Feeding

You can encourage feedings both in the hospital and at home by keeping the room dimly lit and your baby lightly dressed in the early days. After all, your baby has been naked in a dark womb for many months. Bright lights often cause babies to close their eyes and sleep. Also, babies who are dressed and wrapped in blankets are warm, and this warm feeling encourages sleep rather than feeding. Undressing your baby to his diaper and holding his bare body against your bare chest, called skin-to-skin contact, stimulates babies for feedings. Ten minutes of skin-to-skin contact can help wake a sleepy baby.

Feeding Cues

Babies feed best when they are calm. Your baby will show you he is ready to breastfeed long before he cries. Watch for feeding cues: the baby smacking or licking his lips, putting his fist near his mouth, rooting on a blanket, or episodes of light sleep. These subtle signs "tell you" your baby wants to eat.

"Crying is a late indicator of hunger" (AAP, 2005). If a baby becomes too hungry, he may act frantic. Frantic babies cannot eat—their movements become disorganized, and even their tongue changes positions, so latching is impossible. Feed your baby at the first sign of hunger. If your baby is frantic when it is time to breastfeed, take time to soothe and calm him before latching.

Feeding Styles

There are two types of feeding styles in lactation literature: mother-led and baby-led. Mother-led feeding is guided by the mother's movements: how she positions her baby, supports her breast, and quickly helps her baby latch. In contrast, baby-led feeding is guided by the baby's movements. More attention is given to respecting the baby's instinctive feeding behaviors that help him breastfeed. Baby-led feeding is different from mother-led feeding in that baby-led feeding shifts from control to trust and from "steps" to "allowing."

Read through both types of feeding styles. We encourage you to try baby-led feeding first. Ultimately, select the style that works best for you and your baby.

Baby-led Feeding

Healthy babies are born knowing "how" to breastfeed. This knowledge is contained in your baby's reflexes, movements, and behaviors. Recognizing and accepting your baby's natural behaviors will help him breastfeed. Current research supports the idea that babies instinctively know how to find the breast, latch, and feed. Allowing your baby to proceed through a series of predictable movements in his own time will facilitate a successful breastfeed. This is called "baby-led feeding" and is relatively new in lactation literature (Smillie, 2008). In the following paragraphs, we give you a condensed version of baby-led feeding. For a more detailed explanation, please look at *Breastfeeding Made Simple* by Nancy Mohrbacher and Kathleen Kendall-Tackett.

Baby-led Positioning

To begin baby-led feeding, support your body with pillows, so your back, arms, and neck are comfortable. Place your bare or lightly dressed baby on your bare chest. This skin-to-skin contact will awaken his feeding behaviors. Lean back slightly, so gravity keeps your baby's body touching yours. You can hold your baby's hips against your body, allowing him to freely move his arms as he prepares to feed (**Figure 2.1**). It is this full-body touch that stimulates your baby's feeding behaviors (Colson, Meek, & Hawdon, 2008). In this position, your baby may bob his head, "cycle" his little arms around the breast, sometimes brush the nipple with his hand, and suck his hands. These head, arm, and hand movements help your baby organize himself for coordinated, successful feedings. Also, your baby needs a place to support his feet. This can be accomplished by letting the soles of his feet rest on your lap or a pillow. Swaddling your healthy baby can disrupt his interest in breastfeeding because he cannot use his natural body movements.

Babies who have had extended hospital stays or are born with medical needs may not show these feeding behaviors and will require special consideration. If your baby falls into this category, please continue to see or seek out a breastfeeding helper.

Figure 2.1

Mother is leaning back, so baby's body is fully supported on the mother's body. She is supporting his shoulders and hips.

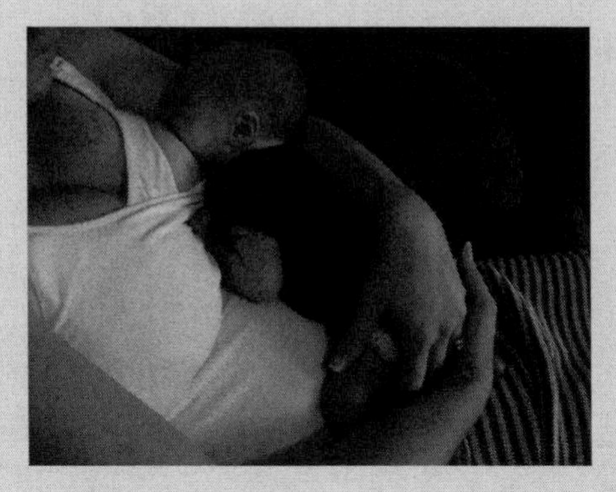

Baby-led Latching

When you and your baby find a comfortable feeding position, you can support your baby's shoulders and neck as necessary to provide stability for latching. Your baby's face will touch your breast as he prepares to feed. Smillie has observed that if a baby's face loses contact with the mother's breast, he is likely to become disorganized and act as though the breast has been removed (Smillie, 2008). **Your baby can achieve the best latch when he approaches the breast chin first.** When the breast is in contact with his chin, this pressure will trigger your baby's mouth to open widely. His head will tip back slightly as he latches. In addition to full body contact, maintaining breast to face contact will help your baby master breastfeeding.

Mother-led Feeding

There are several mother-led breastfeeding positions. You may have learned about these positions in other breastfeeding books or while attending a childbirth or breastfeeding class. Most common is the cradle position, where your baby is held in one arm and feeds on the same breast. You have probably seen this position in photos. It is also the most frequently used position for breastfeeding older babies. Another common position is the cross-cradle position. In this position, the mother has a free hand to shape and support her breast.

If your baby is unable to achieve a good latch in the baby-led feeding style or if you are more comfortable with a structured approach to feeding, you might prefer a mother-led feeding style. However, because we now know a baby's feeding instincts are an important element in the beginning stages of breastfeeding, we need to be mindful of them during mother-led feeding. To respect your baby's instinctive feeding behaviors, we have applied some elements of baby-led feeding to mother-led feeding in the following section. This brings a needed balance to the mother-led style, so the baby's instinctive feeding behaviors are not ignored. For clarity, we have called this **interactive feeding**.

Interactive Positioning

To begin, start with a pillow on your lap to support your baby and bring him to the height of your breast; you should not have to lean forward to breastfeed. As your baby lays across your lap, let his arms hug your breast; do not swaddle your baby. Snuggle him tightly against your body; make sure there are no gaps between your body and his. His shoulders, belly, and hips need to be facing the same direction as his head. His nose, not his lips, will be centered at your nipple, so when he latches, he will slightly tip his head back. Use plenty of pillows to fully support your baby, so his whole body remains in contact with your body. Some mothers use pillows from their bed; some use one of the many commercially available breastfeeding pillows. Use what works best for you. Mothers' shapes are so varied, what worked for your friend may not work for you.

In the cross-cradle hold, you support your breast with the hand on the same side of the body (right breast supported with right hand), while the other hand supports your baby's neck and shoulders, not the back of his head. Hold your breast well behind the areola and out of your baby's way. Your thumb will be on the baby's "nose side," and your fingers on the baby's "chin side." Squeeze the fingers holding the breast together gently, and then pull your breast tissue *back* toward your chest wall, not toward the baby's mouth, to help your nipple protrude more. If you are using the cross-cradle hold, keeping your elbow down will reduce fatigue (**Figures 2.2a & b**). With time, your baby will be able to breastfeed without breast support during the whole feeding.

Figure 2.2a &b

Interactive cross-cradle position: baby's body is in full contact with his mother's body, his face against her breast; mother's left hand supports her left breast, her elbow is down.

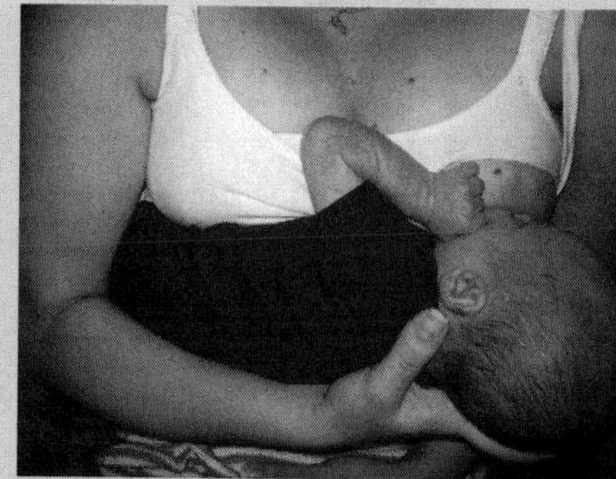

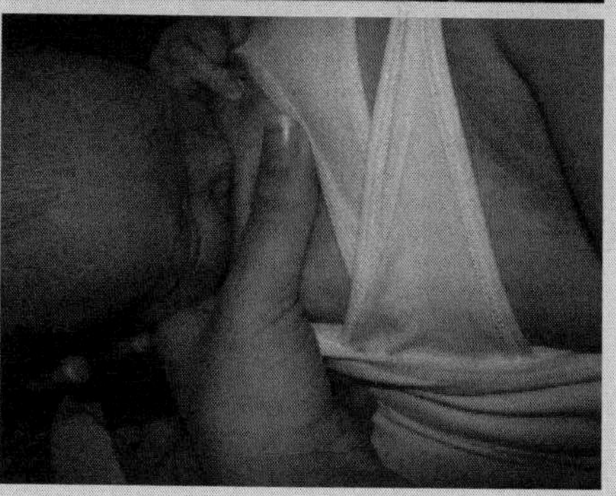

Interactive Latching

In all interactive positions, your baby's nose, not his lips, will be centered at your nipple. It is **not** necessary to brush your nipple across the baby's lips. Your baby latches easier when your breast remains in contact with his face. Instead, your nipple will be touching above your baby's top lip, and your breast will gently rest on his lips and chin, so he can feel your breast on his face. This allows him to latch chin-first, with his head tilted slightly back as in baby-led feeding. Your baby needs to accept more of the areola below the nipple than above it. This helps the breast go deeper into his mouth and allows him to feed more effectively. Babies extract milk from the areola, not the nipple, so a deep latch is important.

Since you are planning to introduce a bottle, you need to pay attention to lip placement. If your baby's lips roll in, the first step in correction is to remove the baby from the breast and relatch. Sometimes lips can be flipped out without relatching the baby. Either way, it is important to be aware of best lip placement, so your baby can mimic this position on a bottle nipple. Babies who roll their lip(s) under while nursing, often do so on a bottle. Lips that roll under while bottle-feeding usually cause the baby to apply pressure with his lips to extract milk, rather than producing a good suck on the bottle.

Checking your baby's lips can be made easier by gently pressing your breast in and away from the baby's mouth, being careful not to disrupt his latch (**Figure 2.3**). You are looking for a lower lip that is rolled outward, called flanged. The top lip will be visible and should not be rolled under. If your baby's lip or lips are rolled under, you can re-latch your baby for a better position, or use a finger to flip the lip out. It is not advised to adjust his lips more than a couple times during a feeding. If you feel your baby's lips do not maintain proper placement during the feed, contact a breastfeeding helper.

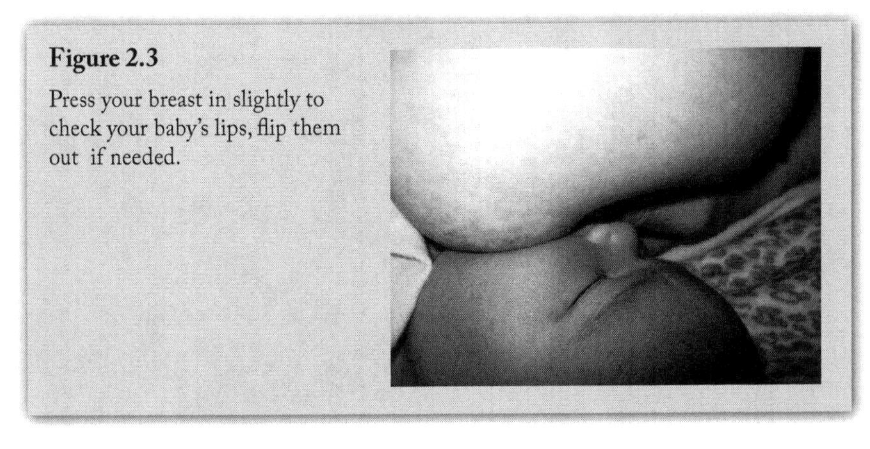

Figure 2.3

Press your breast in slightly to check your baby's lips, flip them out if needed.

The first week or so, you may need to support your breast during the entire feeding if your baby has a hard time staying latched or falls asleep. With time, your baby will be able to breastfeed without needing you to support your breast during the whole feeding.

Outgrowing Careful Positioning

Baby-led feeding is useful during his early days of life when feeding is driven by reflexes and inborn behaviors. Interactive feeding is also helpful in the early days when your baby is learning how the breast feels in his mouth and is mastering a good latch. Regardless of the position you and your baby use, once he has lots of practice, your baby will be a willing participant in any position. You will be able to lift your shirt, and your baby will begin feeding without a thought from you.

Frequency of Feeds

Newborn babies need to eat frequently. Most newborn babies will nurse at least 8-12 times per day, about every 2 hours during the day and every 4 hours at night. If your baby sleeps and does not awaken to eat, you need to help your baby wake up until he does this on his own. Some babies cluster feed, which means the baby will have several feedings close together (every 30 minutes or so), and then take a longer nap. Cluster feeding is okay, too.

Babies should finish breastfeeding at their own pace. Your baby may or may not take the second breast. Babies usually fall asleep after nursing well on one side. At this time, you can burp and change your baby's diaper, then offer the second breast. Breastfeed until your baby falls asleep or pulls away. Start with the second breast at the next feeding.

Evidence of a Good Feeding

When your baby latches, you can check to see if his lower lip is flanged and his upper lip is visible. Your baby will take in the areola as well as the nipple. If he is latching chin first, ideally he will take in more of the areola below the nipple. Babies extract milk from the areola, not the nipple, so a deep latch is important.

Regardless of the position you use, breastfeeding *should not* hurt. However, following the first few days after birth, your baby's latch can make your nipple feel tender or even painful. The pain of the latch is usually from the baby learning how to form your nipple and areola into a teat for feeding. Once the teat is formed, usually within 5-10 seconds, breastfeeding should no longer hurt. After breastfeeding, your nipple should be the same shape as it was before nursing, without creasing or a beveled shape.

This tenderness usually subsides within the first week or so. Once the quantity of your milk increases, usually around day 3-4, you will notice the tenderness subsides as your baby's swallowing increases. If breastfeeding continues to hurt or hurts throughout the feeding, it is important to remove your baby from the breast and re-latch. Get help if the soreness does not improve (Appendix B).

There are specific signs to look for to help you assess if breastfeeding is going well.

- **See**: Your baby's mouth is open wide, bottom lip rolled out, top lip visible, tongue visible under your breast if you gently pull your baby's bottom lip down briefly.
- **Hear**: You may hear swallowing, which becomes more frequent as your body moves from colostrum to milk. When your milk increases in quantity, you will hear one swallow for every one or two sucks. Sometimes, you can see swallowing, too. Your baby's jaw makes short, quick movements at the beginning of a feed to stimulate milk flow, and slow, long movements during a swallow, when the milk is flowing faster.
- **Count**: Your baby will have at least one wet and one poopy diaper per day of life (day 1 = 1 wet and 1 poopy diaper, day 2 = 2 wet and 2 poopy diapers, etc.). After your milk is plentiful, around day 4, the output will increase to 5-6 wet and 2-5 poopy diapers per day, although some babies go more often.
- **Color**: Your baby's first poops will be dark, tar-like stools. If baby is receiving plenty of milk, they should become yellow by day 4 or 5.

Engorgement

Your milk supply increases, or "comes in," around the third or fourth day. During this time, some mothers get engorged: their breasts become warm and uncomfortable. There are several ways to avoid or reduce engorgement. First, try breastfeeding at least every 2 hours. A warm compress or shower before nursing can encourage your milk to flow, while cool compresses between feedings may reduce swelling. In addition, you can ask your physician if Ibuprofen, which reduces swelling and is safe for most nursing mothers, is acceptable for you.

If your breasts are too firm for your baby to latch, there are several ways to soften your breasts. Express just enough milk, with a breast pump or by hand, until your breasts feel soft and allow your baby to latch. There is a commercial product available, Latch Assist, which uses mild suction to help your nipple protrude, allowing your baby to latch more easily. There is also a technique called "Reverse Pressure Softening," where you gently use your fingers to press your areola back toward your chest wall for 1 to 3 minutes before nursing (Cotterman, 2004). This action temporarily moves the swelling back and softens your breast tissue, making it easier for your baby to latch. One website with instructions for this technique is http://www.kellymom.com/bf/concerns/mom/rev_pressure_soft_cotterman.html.

When to Get Help

Sometimes babies are fabulous feeders from birth, others require assistance to figure it out. There are several red-flags that indicate you may need breastfeeding help. These include:

- Breastfeeding hurts throughout an entire feed
- Your nipples become injured
- Your baby cannot remain latched
- Your baby falls asleep or stops nursing immediately after latching
- Your baby does not have enough wet or poopy diapers each day.
- Your baby awakens and cries within ten minutes of a previous feeding
- Your baby does not gain 5.5 - 8.5 ounces or more per week after your milk is in (WHO, 2006;_Bonyata, 2007)

There are breastfeeding helpers in many places. Your local hospital, doctor, or midwife may be able to refer to you to someone, or try the phone book and internet. Breastfeeding helpers have various levels of training, reflected in part in their title. You are welcome to ask your helper what type of training she has received, because often the correct titles are misused. Appendix B defines the different recognized titles breastfeeding helpers may have.

Chapter 3
Understanding Breastfeeding Lingo

Breastfeeding is the natural feeding method for your baby. There are many facets to successful breastfeeding. First and foremost, you and your baby work as a team. The shape of your breast changes as your baby latches and begins to suck. A correct latch and suck action brings a let-down. As your baby feeds, your milk composition changes and increases. This increase in milk is a result of nipple stimulation, which is why avoiding artificial nipples in the beginning is important. To further enhance your understanding of this dynamic, we have highlighted the important aspects of breastfeeding that we will later apply to bottle-feeding.

Mom's Breast

The shape of a mother's breast is very different than its shape when her baby breastfeeds.

- The nipple stretches 2-3 times its resting length, reaching toward the back of the baby's mouth between the hard and soft palate (Nowak, Smith, & Erenberg, 1995). Stretching is sometimes called expanding.
- Areolas can be any size, but a baby will latch well beyond the nipple onto the areola for milk to flow. Sucking on the nipple alone does not produce milk.
- A mother can help her baby achieve a deep latch by supporting her breast, so the baby can take in a large amount of breast tissue beyond the nipple (**Figure 3.1**).

Figure 3.1

Create a deep latch by gently squeezing the breast and pulling back toward your chest wall.

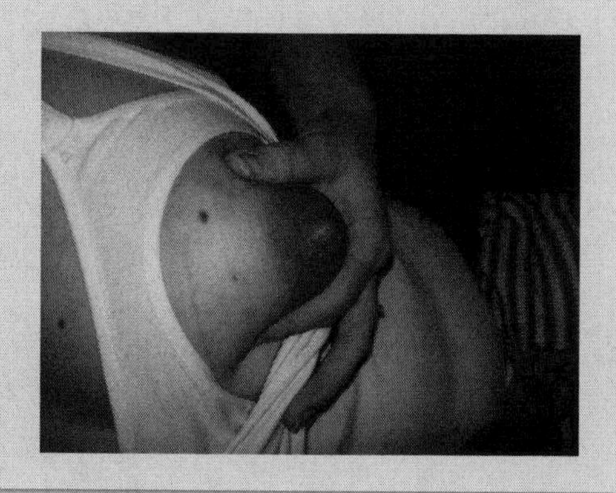

- The diameter of the nipple is reduced 73 ± 5% during the swallow portion of the suck-swallow cycle (Nowak, Smith, & Erenberg, 1994).
- After a baby breastfeeds, the nipple should be the same shape as before the feed began.

Let-downs

Around the fourth day after the baby's birth, the milk supply is more plentiful and many mothers begin to feel their let-down, often described as a tingling sensation. Don't worry if you do not feel this tingling sensation; some mothers never feel a let-down.

Babies usually begin breastfeeding with rapid, short sucks, referred to as non-nutritive sucking (sometimes called flutter sucking). During this time, the baby shapes the nipple and areola into a teat for milk removal. This rapid sucking provides stimulation of the nipples, which causes the milk-ejection reflex, or let-down, and milk starts flowing (Mizuno & Uedo, 2006).

You know your breasts have let-down when your baby's suck changes from rapid, shallow sucks to slow, long sucks, called nutritive sucking. You will probably hear swallowing: one swallow for every one or two sucks.

It is common for your breasts to have several let-downs within one feeding (Geddes, 2009). Your baby will suck and swallow through a let-down, pause and rest, and begin the suck-swallow pattern again with a subsequent let-down.

When your baby feeds on one breast, it is common for the other breast to have let-downs and milk leakage. You will learn how to collect this milk in Chapter 4.

Milk Composition

Breastmilk has two parts: foremilk and hindmilk. The fat is in the hindmilk. The longer your baby feeds on one breast, the higher in fat the milk is. Milk that is full of fat makes him feel full and helps him poop. A baby's poop will usually be yellow when he receives enough fat; it may be green if he does not receive enough fat-rich hindmilk. Green poop indicates he has not nursed long enough or has switched breasts too soon.

Milk Supply

When a mother lets her baby breastfeed as often as the baby wants to suck, it helps ensure a plentiful milk supply. The amount of milk your baby takes while breastfeeding tells your breasts how much milk to produce. This is one of the reasons mothers need to wait 3-4 weeks before introducing a bottle. The more your baby breastfeeds, the better your milk supply will be. This is called supply and demand.

For every bottle your baby receives *without* you pumping your breasts, your body learns to stop producing that many ounces for that particular feeding. To maintain a full milk supply, every time your baby drinks from the bottle, you need to pump your breasts.

Breastfeeding Suck

So what does a *breastfeeding suck* look like? Several things work together to make a good suck. When a baby breastfeeds, we look for:

- Interest the baby: Your baby will be calm. He may be searching for a nipple with his mouth, called rooting.
- Maintain a wide latch: Make sure your baby's mouth opens widely, accepting your nipple and a portion of your areola.
- Position of tongue: Your baby's tongue stays on top of the bottom gum ridge, and the sides of the tongue cradle the nipple. A wave-like motion is visible under the baby's chin during swallowing.
- Lips: The top lip is visible, bottom lip is flipped outward, and both rest gently on the areola.
- Effortless swallow: After a let-down, the baby has a rhythmic swallow pattern, swallowing after every one or two sucks, resting in between let-downs.

Growth Spurt

It is common for babies to breastfeed more often for 2 or 3 days at a time to increase the mother's milk supply. This is referred to as a growth spurt or frequency days.

Growth spurts often occur when the baby is 2 or 3 weeks old, and again at 6 weeks and 3 months (La Leche League International, 2004). Allowing the baby to nurse more often increases the quantity of breastmilk available to the baby. Not allowing the baby to breastfeed frequently or offering a supplement instead of nursing more, tells the mother's body to maintain the current production instead of making more milk, which leads to an inadequate supply later on.

The six-week growth spurt often coincides with the mother's breasts returning to a normal, less-full feeling, and the baby's stooling pattern changing from several bowel movements a day to several days between bowel movements (La Leche League International, 2004). When these normal events occur together, they are often misinterpreted by mothers as an insufficient milk supply. If your breasts stop leaking and feel soft again, and your baby wants to eat more often, this does not mean you don't have enough milk. These events are normal. Do not misinterpret them as a low milk supply.

Nipple Preference

Babies are little humans who have preferences just like adults. Nipple preference happens when a baby prefers the texture, shape, or flow of one nipple over another. To ensure your baby prefers your nipple, it is important in the early days to let your baby learn to suck on one thing, you. Your nipple is the real-deal. Your breasts feel different than a bottle nipple or a pacifier. It is hard work in the beginning for your baby to learn to feed, and letting your baby master latching, sucking, and swallowing with one nipple (yours) is important. This is one reason researchers say to wait 3 to 4 *weeks* before letting your baby try a bottle nipple or pacifier (Howard et al., 2003). By following the information presented in *Balancing Breast and Bottle*, you will learn how to control nipple preference, so that you can be successful in breast and bottle-feeding.

Often, the terms nipple preference and nipple confusion are used interchangeably by professionals, as well as mothers. Nipple preference is different from nipple confusion. The definition of nipple confusion, in the lactation field, is when a baby cannot remember to change his suck from one type of nipple to another. We have found that some babies are labeled as having nipple confusion when, in fact, they have a disorganized or dysfunctional suck at the breast from birth. The introduction of the bottle is not the cause of nipple confusion for these babies. They are born without a good suck. If this sounds like your baby, please see a professional.

Chapter 4
Choosing and Using a Breast Pump

If you will be separated from your baby for multiple feedings, you will need to collect your milk. This ensures a plentiful milk supply for you and allows your baby to have exclusive breastmilk feedings.

Several decisions must be made before choosing a breast pump. First, you must decide if you will rent or purchase a pump. Second, you will need to determine the best pump choice for your specific situation, keeping in mind that pumps are not created equal. Pumps differ in effectiveness and fit. After you find the best pump for you, you will need to learn ways to pump efficiently. Also, pumping will provide an opportunity to learn about your milk and how your breasts let-down.

Unexpected Collecting

Many mothers returning to work full-time begin storing milk ahead of time. Some begin collecting and saving milk as early as a week after the baby's birth, while others wait until 3 or 4 weeks before returning to work. This is referred to as stockpiling. Stockpiling your milk is further discussed in Chapter 11.

There are several ways to collect your milk. When you breastfeed your baby and have a let-down, does your opposite breast leak? Often mothers will let this milk soak into a nursing pad worn inside the bra or onto a burp rag. But wait! This milk can be collected and saved for a future feeding. It is possible to build a great supply without even pumping. One mother collected her leaking milk during breastfeeding sessions and saved 50 six-ounce containers (300 ounces) of milk in two months without even pumping. That equates to 100-150 feedings. Wow!

If your let-down is a steady drip, a bottle held under the opposite breast might be the perfect container (**Figure 4.1**). If your milk sprays rather than drips, a better container might be a clean yogurt container, small bowl, or your breast pump flange and collection bottle.

Another way to collect your dripping milk is with a product on the market called a Milk-Saver that is worn inside the bra on the opposite breast during a feeding (**Figure 4.2**). Dripping milk can be collected in the reservoir or a milk storage bag can be attached. This product is held in place with your bra, so both your hands are "free" to help your baby breastfeed. Since your breasts are likely to leak while breastfeeding, this is a great way to get a head start on saving milk.

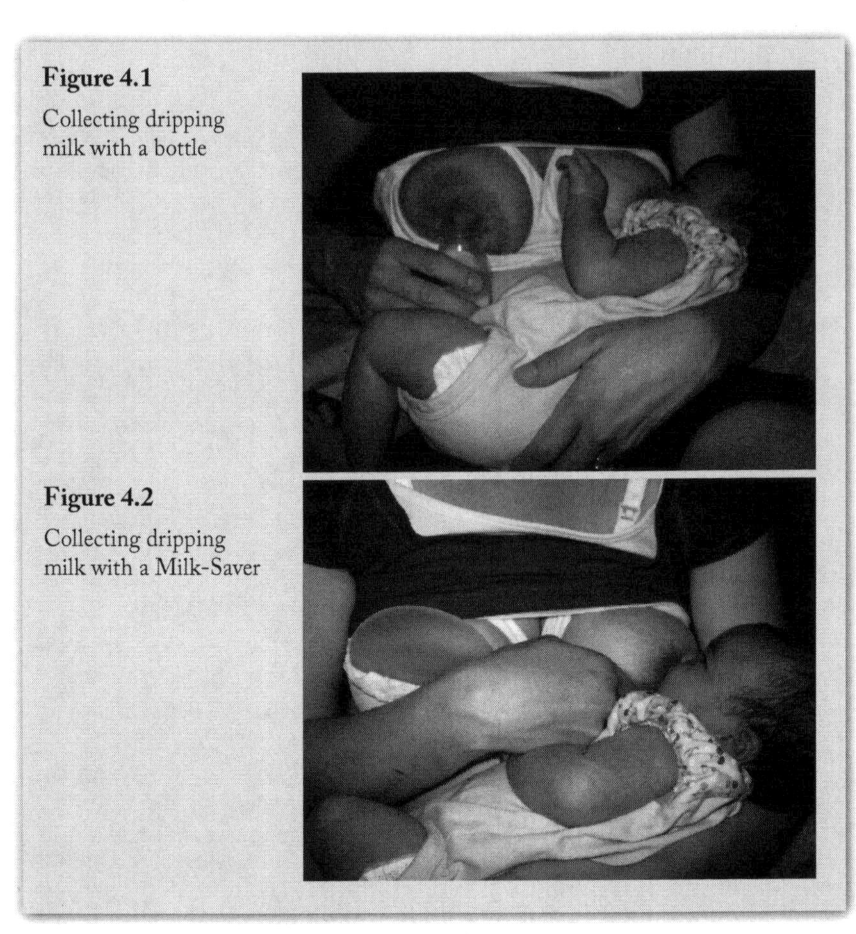

Figure 4.1
Collecting dripping milk with a bottle

Figure 4.2
Collecting dripping milk with a Milk-Saver

Choosing a Breast Pump

It is important to choose the best pump for your situation. Mothers who plan to express their milk occasionally can successfully express by hand (manually) or with a hand-held, non-electric breast pump. For further information on manual expression, refer to *The Womanly Art of Breastfeeding* or your comprehensive breastfeeding book. A hand pump costs around $30-40 US dollars.

The next step up is an electric breast pump that cycles 40 times per minute. This is considered a mid-level pump for a mother who pumps 2-3 times per week. These pumps are often single (pump one breast at a time) rather than double (pump both breasts at the same time). The slower cycling requires pumping for a longer amount of time to yield the same quantity of milk as a higher-grade pump. These pumps are more effective when a mother elicits a let-down before pumping. They are generally considered ideal for part-time use, rather than daily use. This grade of breast pump cannot be used to establish a milk supply. In other words, if you purchase this type of breast pump before your baby's birth and find your baby has difficulty breastfeeding in the early days, you will need to rent or purchase a higher-quality pump to establish your supply.

Within the mid-level category of breast pumps, some brands cycle less than 40 times per minute. These brands should be avoided. Slow cycling causes a less-than-normal amount of milk to be expressed. Most mothers eventually lose their milk supply over time with slow-cycling pumps.

Mothers who will miss more than one feeding daily are most successful when they choose a high-quality, fully automatic, double-electric breast pump to buy or to rent. Using a breast pump that cycles 48-60 times per minute, the same pace that a baby usually sucks, will help you sustain your milk supply and is generally considered the best choice for mothers employed fulltime outside the home. A high quality breast pump is a one-time purchase of $160-$380 US dollars. This is a huge savings compared to the cost of formula. For example, if a baby drinks 32 ounces of breastmilk a day and formula costs between 6.2¢ and 29¢ per ounce, this would mean a cost per month of $64-$288. A high quality pump would be paid for within 1 to 3 months.

New or Used

Most breast pumps are considered "single-user items," which means it is not safe to share or buy a previously used breast pump. The US Food and Drug Administration states, "You should never buy a used breast pump or share a breast pump" (FDA, 2009).

The exceptions are *rental* breast pumps and breast pumps that specify "multiple-user." The user buys a new collection kit of tubing and bottles when using a multiple-user pump. These pumps have a filter to remove pollutants. They pull air away from the bottles toward the pump, so the expressed milk is not at risk for contamination. In most other types of breast pumps, the air flows from the pump motor toward the bottles. Even if a mother purchases a new collection kit for a used single-user pump, there is a risk of bacteria and germs in the motor being "pushed" toward the milk.

When you purchase a new pump, you have the advantage of knowing and feeling how effective your pump is straight out of the box. This knowledge is important. A few weeks or months down the road, if your pump feels less effective, you will know it is time to change the filters or membranes or troubleshoot another problem. If you use your breast pump with subsequent children, you will know if your pump is working at full capacity without having to automatically purchase a new pump with every child.

Breast-Pump Packaging

It can be hard to tell the difference between a high-grade breast-pump and a slow-cycling breast pump by reading the packaging. Most breast-pump manufacturers claim their pumps are fully automatic and for daily use, though their product specifications (cycles and vacuum) reflect the opposite. Similar to bottle-nipple packaging, many breast-pump packages state their brand is "most like breastfeeding" or the "best choice."

Before buying a pump, consider calling the product company's toll-free number to ask for product specifications. Some of this information may not be on the breast pump box. Since breast pumps are a single-user item, you will not be able to return or exchange a breast pump if you buy the wrong one by mistake. When in doubt, call before you purchase.

There are several elements to look for in a high quality pump.

- Double pump—pumps both breasts at the same time, so it can be up to twice as fast (Biagioli, 2003)
- Fully automatic—turn the switch on, and the pump begins, rather than the mother controlling the pumping by squeezing a handle or pressing a lever to regulate the vacuum or the cycles
- Cycles up to 60 times per minute—pumps that cycle less than this, or cycle as fast as the mother controls the lever, often result in a reduced milk supply over time
- Up to 250mmHg—millimeters of Mercury, this measures suction

Another hallmark of a high-quality pump is compression. Pumps with this feature typically are not found on chain-store shelves, and they are quite expensive. However, this component improves milk flow (Alekseev et al., 1998).

Be wary of pump directions (often available for review online) that recommend hand expression to elicit a let-down *before* you begin pumping. This may be an indication of a lesser-quality pump that is perhaps adequate for occasional use, but not ideal for daily use.

Proper Fit

It is important that your pump flange fits properly. The flange is the part of the breast pump that is held to your breast as you pump. Large breasts do not equal large flanges; the nipple diameter determines the flange size you need. Your nipple should move freely in the flange "tunnel" while pumping. If your nipple rubs the flange or fits tightly, you need to purchase a larger size flange. Likewise, if the flange does not form an airtight seal or if a good portion of your breast tissue is pulled into the flange (in addition to your nipple), use a reducing insert or purchase a smaller flange. Some breast pump companies have multiple flanges to choose from—another consideration in choosing your breast pump. For more information about multiple flange sizes, visit our website www.breastandbottlefeeding.com.

Tips for Optimal Use of Your Breast Pump

Your pump will work most effectively when you remember the tips in Table 1.

Table 1. Tips for Optimal Use of Your Breast Pump

Small bottles	Use empty 4-ounce containers for each pumping session. If your bottles become full during a single session, pour collected milk into another container. Adjust the vacuum down as the bottles fill.
Filter or membrane—the piece between the flange and bottle	Keep extra filters or membranes on hand. Store a pair *with* your breast pump, so if you need this piece while outside your home, you have it.
Power supply	If you use your breast pump with batteries, replace or recharge the batteries every couple days. Plan to keep extra batteries stored with your breast pump, just in case you need them.
Dry tubing between collection kit and pump motor	If you notice moisture or milk in the pump tubing after you pump, remove the tubing from the flanges, and then let the pump continue to run. The air movement through the tubing will cause the moisture to evaporate within a couple of minutes.

Your Milk

The first time you pump your milk do not be surprised if you only express a small quantity. Your body must learn to respond to the pump. Over time your body will be able to express more milk. The time it takes to have a let-down, also called milk ejection, is different between breastfeeding and pumping. On average, it takes 52-60 seconds to elicit milk ejection when breastfeeding (Kent, Ramsay, Doherty, Larsson & Hartmann, 2003) and over 3 minutes of pumping until ejection occurs (Mitoulas, Lai, Gurrin, Larsson & Hartmann, 2002). Mitoulas and colleagues (2002) reported this number in seconds as 103.2 ±89.2. When pumping, it is normal for one breast to produce more milk than the other. Also, one breast might drip while the other sprays—that is okay. Using a breast pump is not a reflection of how much milk your baby receives; your baby's suck is more effective than your pump.

When you are pumping, you might notice your milk is different colors at different times of the day, and often different within one pumping session. Sometimes it may look clear or watery, yellow or white, or many shades in between. This is normal. This color variation is a change in the fat content of your milk. The foods you eat can also tint the color of your milk. For example, eating beets can make your milk look reddish, and eating lots of green vegetables can make your milk look greenish. Again, this is normal. You can feed your baby, even when your milk is tinted.

Achieving multiple let-downs while you pump allows you to collect more milk. Stimulating multiple let-downs can be accomplished with breast massage. Breast massage uses motions similar to a breast self-exam. You will want to massage your breasts before you begin pumping, and also while you pump. Massage your breasts by placing your fingers toward the outside of your breast, press gently and make circular motions. Repeat this motion around your breast, working toward the nipple. A second massage technique is to lightly slide your fingertips from the outside of the breasts toward the nipple, like you are outlining the spokes of a wheel from the rim toward the center. When you are pumping with a double pump, brace the pump flanges with one arm, so your free hand can massage your breasts alternately. Not only will massaging your breasts during pumping increase your yield, it will also help you prevent plugged ducts (Riordan, 2010).

Another idea to stimulate your let-down is listening to relaxing music while nursing your baby, and then listening to the same music while pumping. Smelling your baby's blanket or a clothing item and looking at your baby's picture may help you enlist your senses to achieve faster let-downs. A commercial product available is the *"Sense Memory Method of Milk Expression,"* a CD with music and baby sounds to help mothers let-down when pumping. Some breast pumps have a recording device that allows mothers to record their baby's sounds and replay while pumping.

Some mothers practice pumping twice a day, usually in the morning, when the milk supply is highest. Practicing each day will help your breasts learn to let-down to the stimulation of the pump. Storing your milk is discussed in Chapter 11.

Now that you have your pump and are familiar with the pieces, it is time for you to practice with your pump and for your baby to practice with a bottle, so pump some milk and let's get started.

SECTION 2
Artificial Nipples

Chapter 5
Language of Bottles

When discussing bottles, it seems every brand has a unique terminology for their bottles. Thankfully, there are some universal terms we will now explore, so we are all speaking the same "language."

Parts of a Bottle

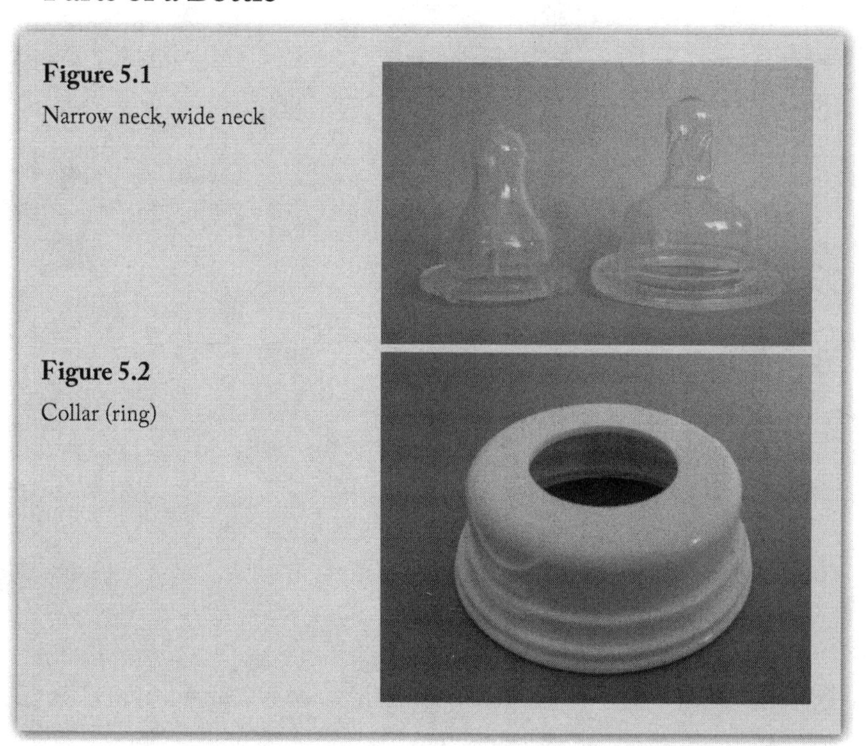

Figure 5.1
Narrow neck, wide neck

Figure 5.2
Collar (ring)

Most bottles have a nipple and a collar (**Figures 5.1** and **5.2**). Bottle nipples come in two general sizes: **narrow** (sometimes called standard) and **wide** neck. Narrow-neck bottle nipples have a smaller base, and they tend to fit most narrow-neck bottles. Wide-neck bottles have a wider base and work with fatter bottles.

The **collar** is the ring the nipple fits into. The collar then screws onto the bottle. Some collars are interchangeable with various brands of nipples and bottles, while some are not.

Parts of a Nipple

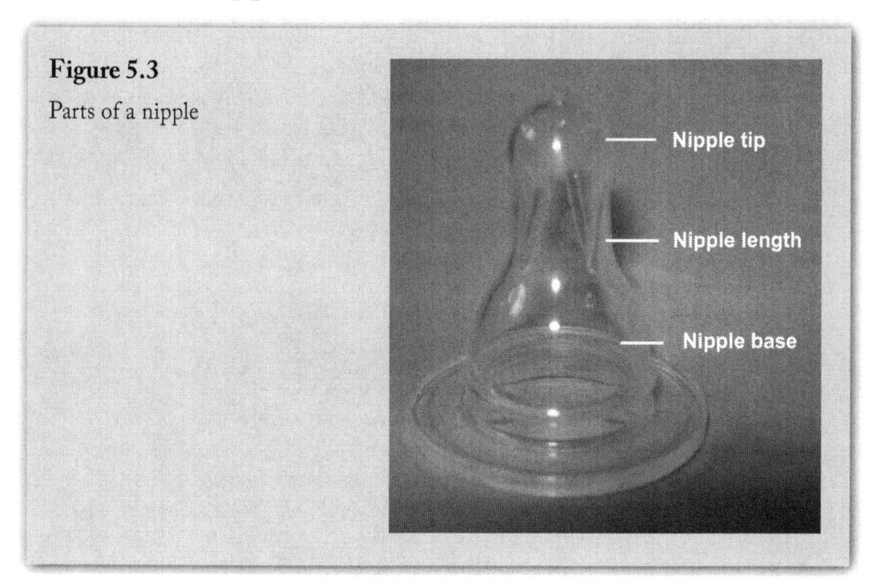

Figure 5.3
Parts of a nipple

Nipples have three parts (**Figure 5.3**). The **nipple tip** is the end where the milk flows out. The **nipple length** is the part of the nipple that is in contact with the baby's tongue. Nipple lengths vary; some are short and some are long. The **nipple base** is the lower part of the nipple. This part is like a mother's areola—the baby's lips are intended to rest gently on a portion of the nipple base. While nipple shapes may vary greatly, every bottle nipple has these three elements.

Other Common Terms

Vent is another bottle term. The vent, or venting system, allows air pressure in the bottle to equalize as the baby sucks. This can help prevent the baby from swallowing air. Some babies do fine with a nipple or feeding system that does not have a venting system; most babies naturally "vent" when they burp.

Even so, many bottle systems attempt to control air pressure. Some nipples, such as the Nuk® and Soothie have a vented nipple; there is a hole cut into the nipple base. Many nipples do not have a vent. Instead, the bottle itself or the bottle collar has a venting system. Dr. Brown's, Ventaire®, and

Born Free™ have a bottle with a venting mechanism. Munchkin®'s collar contains the venting system. Other feeding systems, such as Playtex® Drop-ins™ and Kiinde™, have a collapsing liner instead of a venting system. The venting system is often associated with claims of reducing gas and colic. In our practice, we have found that when healthy babies without reflux issues have a good mouth placement and seal on a bottle nipple, along with a slow, rhythmic swallow pattern, gas and colic are reduced regardless of the feeding system.

Flow is a bottle-nipple term, sometimes called size or flow-rate. This refers to how fast the milk comes out of the nipple. There are generally three flow rates to choose from: slow, medium, and fast. The flow will be printed on the package, but it is also usually printed on the bottle nipple, towards the nipple base.

The rate of flow will influence your baby's coordination while bottle-feeding. Most babies begin with a slow nipple, called "size 1," "slow-flow," or "newborn" nipple. Not all slow-flow nipples are created equal. The flow rate varies among and within bottle-nipple brands. We have tested and categorized various brands of slow flow nipples as very-slow, medium-slow, and fast-slow. This list is found in Appendix C.

The rate of flow is important. We have observed that babies become fussy and/or disinterested in feeding when a nipple flows too slowly, and that babies choke, gag, and/or cry when a nipple flows too quickly. Based on these observations, we suggest that bottle nipples with flow rates under .3mL are too slow for most babies, while flows over .8mL are too fast for others.

Some bottle nipples are packaged as "no-drip" nipples. This means that when the bottle nipple is tipped down, the nipple will not leak. Many nipples become no-drip nipples, even though they are not packaged as such. Inverting a bottle nipple for 5 seconds allows the air pressure in the bottle to equalize, making many nipples stop dripping.

Dripping does not indicate how fast a nipple flows, though. Just because a bottle nipple is no-drip does not mean that the milk will flow more slowly when a baby sucks on it. Dripping is not a clear indicator of milk flow.

Texture is a term used to describe the feel of the nipple. Bottle companies often give a nod to texture by putting statements on their packaging, such as "just like mom." Otherwise, there is no indication of the nipple texture. In the past, nipple texture has not been a consideration in selecting a nipple because there was little variation. With recent advances in silicone products, manufacturers have been able to develop a wide range of nipple textures with some of the newer nipples being extra soft. An extra soft nipple sounds ideal because most breasts have a soft texture once the milk supply regulates. However, while the breast feels soft to the touch, it provides resistance when squeezed due to the internal structure of the breast. This density helps the breast maintain its shape, aiding the baby's mouth placement during latch. If the bottle nipple texture is too soft, the baby's lips may compress the nipple and roll inward because most bottle nipples do not provide resistance like the breast.

An **orthodontic** nipple differs from other nipple shapes in that it resembles a tube of lipstick. The nipple tip is bulbous on one side with a flat slope on the other.

Feeding system refers to using the same brand of bottle nipple, bottle, and collar. Many mothers wonder if it is okay to buy a whole feeding system. We suggest you purchase one bottle or package of replacement nipples before buying a whole feeding system. Every baby sucks differently, which is why we cannot suggest that one nipple is "best," although we have found that narrow neck nipples often produce a better latch than wide neck nipples. After you find the best nipple for your baby, then it is safe to buy a feeding system.

Chapter 6
Getting Started

Bottle introduction can seem scary. It is a taboo subject. You have probably read that you need to avoid or limit the use of bottles. This is not practical in every situation, particularly when a mother will be employed outside the home. Suggestions on when to introduce a bottle and who should introduce it are often wrapped in old wives' tales and misinterpreted as fact. Let's take a realistic look at bottle use, including the "when's and who's" of introduction and the supplies and positioning techniques that will be helpful.

Preferred Age of Baby

The question of when to introduce a bottle is a delicate balance of making sure you have waited long enough to establish breastfeeding, but not so long that your baby is unwilling to accept an artificial nipple. A perfect time to help your baby explore feedings with a bottle is at 3-4 weeks of age. You have patiently helped your baby learn to breastfeed and have asked for help when needed. You know how to express your milk, and you know your baby needs your breastmilk in the bottle. *Now* you are ready to learn about introducing a bottle.

At 3-4 weeks of age, your baby is young enough not to fight the idea of sucking on an object other than you. It is possible to coax a baby older than 4 weeks of age to accept a bottle, but we feel the potential battle and worry about how your baby is going to eat while you are away is not worth the wait. Waiting to introduce a bottle until just prior to returning to work, as suggested in various breastfeeding books, can end in tears and frustration for you, your baby, and your caregiver because your baby may have developed a preference for your breast. We suggest a kinder, gentler approach to introducing the bottle, hopefully eliminating any panic and sadness.

In *Nursing Mother, Working Mother*, Gale Pryor (1997, p. 112) writes, "...babies who first try the bottle after two months of age are often intractable in their preference for the breast," meaning a baby this old will often reject the bottle nipple. Likewise, in *The Whole Parenting Guide*, the authors suggest that older babies may develop "*nipple chauvinism* in which a baby is definitely *not* confused, and wants *only* mother's breast" (Reder, Catalfo & Renfrow Hamilton, 1999, p. 60). We agree and add that past 4 weeks old is the age of bottle nipple resistance for most babies.

An exception for bottle introduction is when a mother will be returning to work or school before the typical six-week maternity leave. If a mother is returning to school when her baby is 3 weeks old, introducing the bottle at 2 weeks of age is acceptable. Likewise, if a mother is returning to work when her baby is 4 weeks old, introducing the bottle by 3 weeks is preferred. Create at least 1 week of practice time, so you and your baby feel ready.

Who Introduces the Bottle

Many texts suggest having a caregiver other than the mother introduce a bottle to help avoid nipple confusion. We dispute that nipple confusion is linked to the person introducing a bottle. As you will read in future chapters, nipple confusion can be caused by poor nipple selection and feeding techniques that do not support breastfeeding. Instead of having someone else introduce a bottle to your baby, we recommend that you introduce the bottle.

You, the mother, are the one who is intimately acquainted with your baby's suck. You know what your baby's lips look like when he feeds, how widely he naturally latches on your breast, and how long your let-downs last. You are the most equipped person to choose a bottle nipple for your baby. Once you have chosen the best nipple for your baby, you can then teach another adult how to bottle-feed your baby to mimic breastfeeding as closely as possible.

Which Shapes to Try First

Different nipple shapes work with different babies. You may have a variety of nipple shapes at home. If you want to try the nipples you have on hand first, be certain they are new, recently purchased nipples. Nipples saved from a sibling or received "used" from a friend often deteriorate over time, and the flow may be too fast. Also, if you received bottles as a gift, double check the flow by removing the nipple from the collar and reading the base of the nipple to determine what size nipple it is.

Sometimes a mother will start from scratch and need to purchase a couple of nipples for her baby. We typically begin with these shapes (**Figure 6.1**).

Figure 6.1
Initial shapes to try

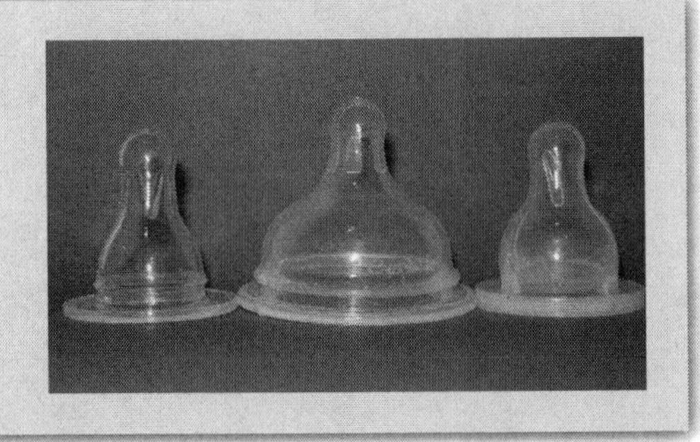

These shapes are not "better" than others, but they do provide a nice transition from tip to base. They also allow for observation of the baby sucking on a narrow-neck nipple, as well as a wide-neck nipple.

Wide-neck nipples are a popular choice for breastfed babies. They are usually advertised as a better choice than narrow-neck nipples. Wide-neck nipples are often recommended as a first choice in breastfeeding books. To the contrary, we disagree. We have not found that wide-neck nipples are a better choice for every baby, but that the scale tips in favor of narrow-neck nipples, with the exception of babies with tongue tie. See p. 77 for more information.

The First-Bottle Introduction

Plan to introduce the bottle during a happy, peaceful time of day. For many families, morning works best. Choose a snack-time, which means your baby will use the bottle between his typical breastfeeding meals. It is important that your baby is neither full nor hungry when the bottle is introduced.

When you are ready to choose a nipple for your baby, described in the following chapter, you will need 2-3 ounces of expressed, warm milk. If you are trying more than one brand of bottle and the nipples are not interchangeable, it may be helpful to put ½-1 ounce of milk in each bottle. Have your supplies lined up, ready to use.

Finding a Free Hand

While your baby is learning to bottle-feed, it might seem you need an extra hand. Typically, one arm cradles the baby while the other hand holds the bottle. While your baby is learning, you will probably need another hand to evaluate and adjust your baby's mouth placement. While we cannot help you grow an extra arm, we do know how to free up a hand (**Figure 6.2**).

Figure 6.2

Baby supported on leg, one hand holds the bottle, the other is free

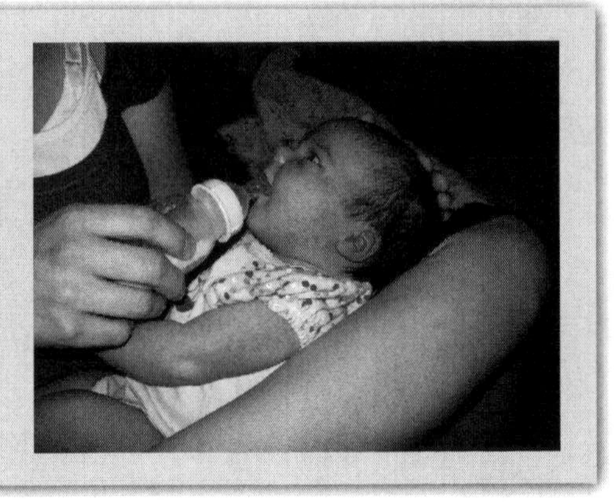

Sitting with your legs crossed, possibly with a pillow over your knee, let your baby lie in a semi-upright position facing you. Your leg, or pillow, will be your extra arm, cradling and supporting your baby. One of your hands will offer the bottle, while the other hand is free to adjust your baby's lips, take a peek at tongue position by pulling the lip down, and any other minor adjustments your baby needs, which you will learn about in the next chapter. This position gives you an unobstructed view for evaluating your baby's suck. Once you have found the best nipple for your baby, you can switch to a more natural feeding position, cradling your baby in your arm.

Dripping and Breastfeeding

To make bottle-feeding more like breastfeeding, it is important that the bottle is not dripping into the baby's mouth before he begins sucking. Test your bottle nipple. Does it stop dripping after you aim the nipple tip down for a few seconds? If the answer is yes, let it equalize in pressure and stop dripping before you offer it to your baby. If the answer is no and the bottle continues to drip, hold the bottle so the milk does not reach the nipple tip. Once your baby begins to suck, tip the bottle, so the milk reaches the nipple tip. Both of these techniques will help your baby control the flow at the beginning of a feed, making bottle-feeding more like breastfeeding. This is discussed more in depth in Chapter 8, *Evaluating Bottle-feeding Difficulties*.

Chapter 7
Selection Made SIMPLE

Maintaining and protecting your breastfeeding relationship is necessary, so it is key that the nipple you select allows your baby to switch between breast and bottle easily. Since breastfeeding is the natural feeding method, we apply the qualities of breastfeeding, explored in Chapter 3, to bottle-feeding. We will look at the characteristics of various bottle nipples and your baby's response to help you choose the best nipple for your baby.

There are specific steps in selecting a bottle nipple for a breastfed baby. To begin, we examine the components of a nipple, including the flow, shape, and texture. Next, we consider the baby's temperament and willingness to feed. Evaluating the baby's mouth placement and suck follows. Lastly, we listen to the baby's swallowing pattern. We have developed a method that describes these steps of bottle introduction and have termed it the SIMPLE Method.

SIMPLE Method

The SIMPLE Method is an acronym that identifies the various steps in choosing a bottle nipple for a breastfed baby. Each letter stands for a phrase describing one step of bottle introduction. Every step is important in determining the best bottle nipple for your baby.

S **Select a nipple**: Start with a slow-flow nipple that gradually flares from length to base and has an appropriate texture.

I **Interest the baby**: Beginning when your baby is 3-4 weeks of age, introduce the bottle to your baby when he is alert and calm. Allow him to latch onto a bottle nipple that is not dripping.

M **Maintain a wide latch**: Make sure your baby's mouth is widely open, accepting the nipple length in addition to a portion of the nipple base.

P **Position of tongue**: Check that your baby's tongue stays over bottom gum ridge, with the sides cupping the nipple, moving in a wave-like motion visible under your baby's chin during swallowing.

L **Lips**: Make sure your baby's lips stay flanged, which means the top lip is visible and the bottom lip flips outward. Both lips should gently rest on a portion of the nipple base. After your baby latches onto the bottle nipple, adjust your baby's lips.

E **Effortless swallow**: Listen for a rhythmic swallow pattern. Your baby should swallow after every one or two sucks, without gulping or gagging.

Now that you have been introduced to the SIMPLE Method, let's explore each step in detail and see how bottle-feeding can be related to breastfeeding. Beginning with "Select a nipple," we will move through each step, highlighting a successful nipple choice.

Select a Nipple

Nipple selection begins with three considerations: flow, shape, and texture. Evaluate the flow, nipple shape, and nipple texture before offering a bottle nipple to your baby.

The rate of **flow** will influence your baby's coordination while bottle-feeding. Most breastfed babies begin with a "size 1" or "slow-flow" nipple. This was discussed in detail in the previous chapter, *The Language of Bottles.* The **shape** of the bottle nipple determines mouth placement. When your baby breastfeeds, your nipple reaches toward the back of the baby's mouth, and your baby's mouth accepts the nipple and areola. When your baby bottle-feeds, the nipple length needs to approximate a similar placement, reaching toward the back of your baby's mouth. Your baby's lips should be open, accepting a portion of the nipple base. When you look at a bottle nipple, consider how the length transitions to the base. A gradual transition between the nipple length and base typically provides better mouth placement (**Figures 7.1** and **7.2**).

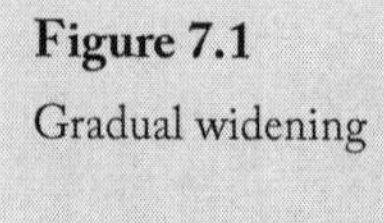

Figure 7.1
Gradual widening

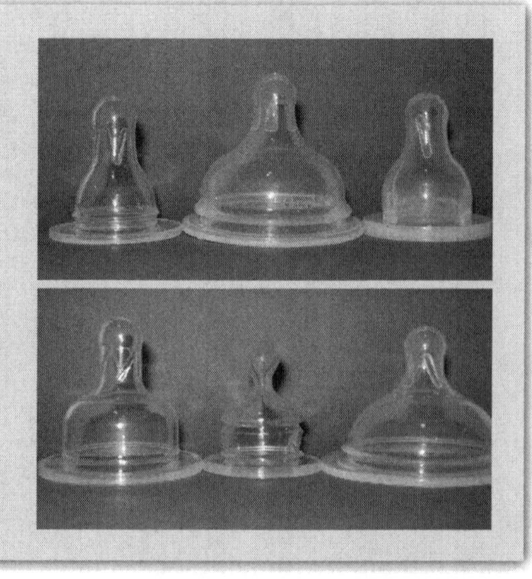

Figure 7.2
Abrupt widening

In selecting a nipple, you must also consider **texture.** Every mother's breast has a unique texture. Luckily, there is a wide selection of bottle nipple textures on the market, ranging from hard and stiff to soft and squishy. Nipples that are too firm in texture can make the baby's mouth tired, stretch the lips too tightly, or cause the baby to slide to the tip. Nipples that are extra soft in texture will likely collapse as the baby applies pressure, cause the lips to roll in, and may also cause the baby to slide to the tip. These problems can occur whether the nipple shape is abrupt or gradual.

Interest Baby

When you breastfeed your baby, he is interested in feeding and concentrating on the task at hand. Your baby latches best when he is calm, because his tongue is in the correct position to accept the nipple. Your baby roots or searches for your nipple by widely opening his mouth. These same behaviors are applied when we interest a baby in latching onto a bottle.

To introduce a bottle to your baby, choose a time when he is happy and alert. Rest the bottle above your baby's top lip or gently stroke his lips with the bottle nipple. Let him widely open his mouth, like when he is breastfeeding. Do not push the nipple into your baby's mouth. Let your baby take the nipple in, and then adjust his lips to roll outward like a fish (**Figure 7.3**).

Figure 7.3

Present nipple to baby's lips and let baby open wide

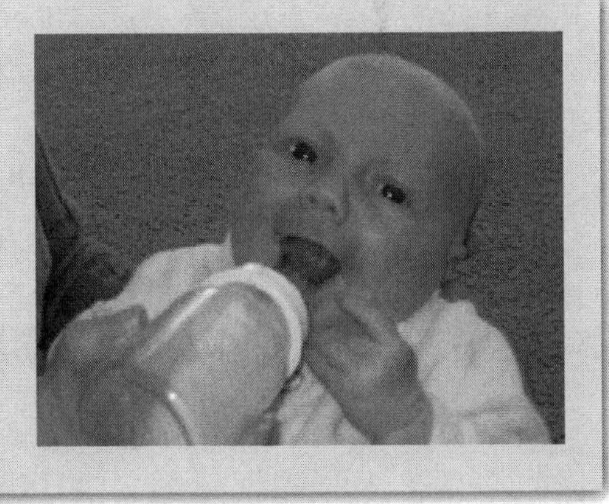

Maintain a Wide Latch

When your baby breastfeeds, you see his mouth widely open to latch. Your baby accepts your nipple and your areola. Your baby's mouth remains widely opened throughout the feeding. When your baby bottle-feeds, we want his mouth position to mimic this.

Your baby's mouth needs to be widely opened, accepting a portion of the nipple base in addition to the nipple length, and he needs to maintain this position throughout the feeding. Some babies achieve good mouth placement on a narrow nipple (**Figure 7.4**). Other babies achieve good mouth placement on a wide nipple (**Figure 7.5**).

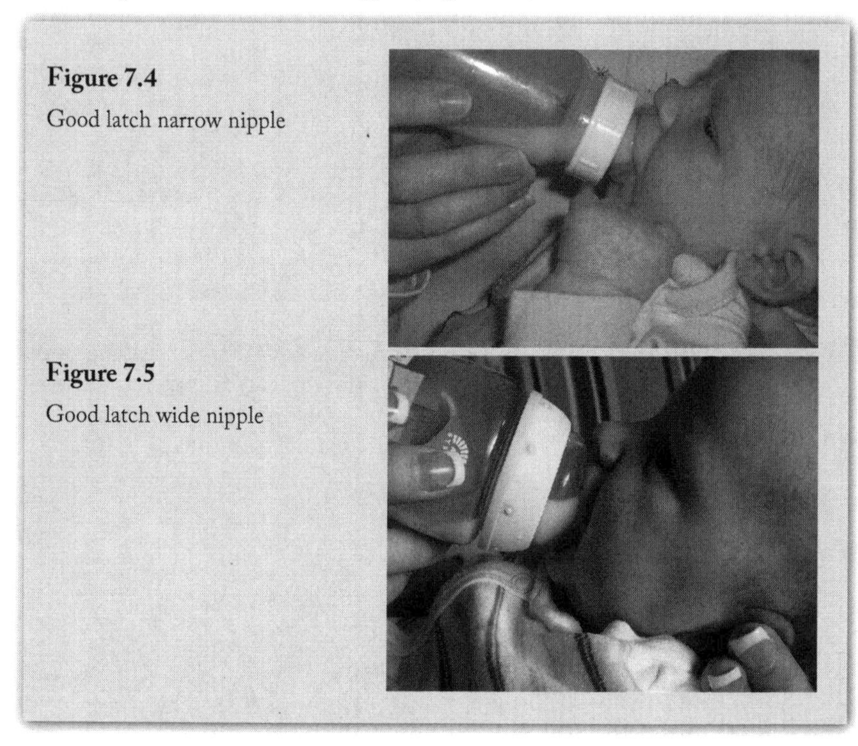

Figure 7.4

Good latch narrow nipple

Figure 7.5

Good latch wide nipple

Position of Tongue

When your baby breastfeeds, you can see that his tongue stays over his bottom gum ridge if you gently pull his bottom lip down. You can also see the sides of the tongue cradling the nipple. When your baby swallows, called nutritive sucking, you will notice a wave-like motion visible under your baby's chin.

The shape of the bottle nipple should allow for normal tongue positioning and movement. You will be able to see your baby's tongue over the gum ridge when you pull the lip down slightly during bottle-feeding (**Figure 7.6**). When you pull the bottle from your baby's mouth, you will see tongue cupping (**Figure 7.7**).

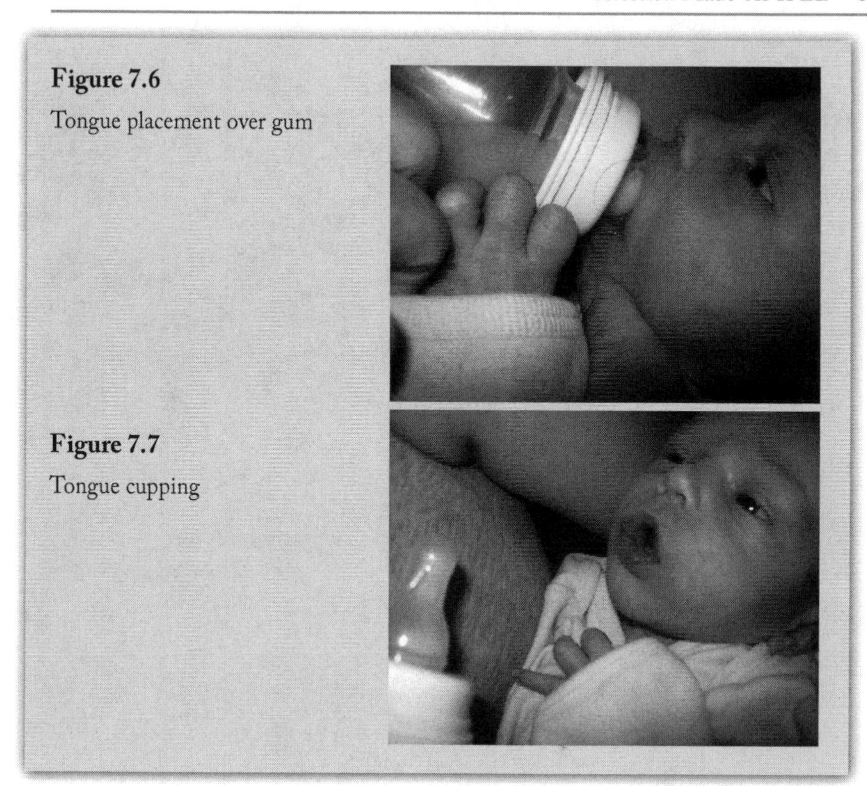

Figure 7.6
Tongue placement over gum

Figure 7.7
Tongue cupping

When a baby sucks correctly, his tongue will move in a wave-like motion when he swallows. This movement is visible under the baby's chin.

Lips

Your baby's lips are flanged during breastfeeding. This means the top is visible and the bottom lip flips outward, sealing on your breast. Your baby's lips gently rest on your areola during breastfeeding. You do not see gaps between your breast and the corners of your baby's mouth. Gaps allow unwanted air into your baby's tummy.

This same lip placement is needed on a bottle nipple. The baby's top lip is visible and his bottom lip rolls outward. The baby's lips are in contact with some of the nipple base, leaving no air gaps between the nipple and the corners of the baby's mouth. The baby's lips gently rest on the nipple base, not on the collar (**Figure 7.8**).

Figure 7.8

Lips resting on a portion of nipple base, not collar

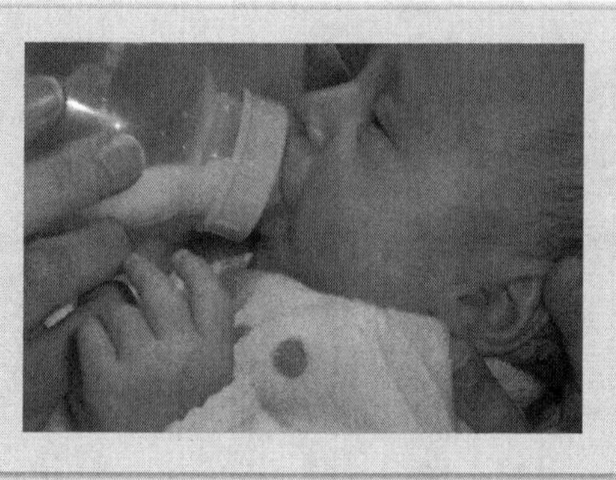

Effortless Swallow

When you begin breastfeeding, your baby suckles without much swallowing to stimulate your let-down. This is called non-nutritive sucking. Once your milk lets-down, your baby has a rhythmic swallow pattern, swallowing after every one or two sucks, resting in between let-downs.

With bottle-feeding, your baby will have a rhythmic swallow pattern, swallowing after every one or two sucks, without gulping or gagging. Most babies suck 20-30 times in row, and then rest. Along with rhythmic swallowing, your baby should look relaxed while bottle-feeding.

As you can see, there are many components that work together in choosing a bottle nipple and introducing it to your baby. You select a nipple according to flow, shape, and texture, and elicit your baby's latch when he is calm and alert. You evaluate how wide his latch is compared with breastfeeding, as well as evaluating the position of his tongue and lips. Finally, you listen for rhythmic swallowing. When all the pieces work together successfully, you have found a good nipple choice for your baby. Congratulations, your nipple selection achieved a suck similar to that of breastfeeding. If it did not, the next chapter highlights common problems and offers suggestions for improvement.

Chapter 8
Evaluating Bottle-Feeding Difficulties

You have learned about the SIMPLE Method and its effectiveness in choosing the best nipple for your baby. Not all babies are textbook babies, and despite your careful consideration and selection, your baby may not be successful on the first nipple you try.

If your baby is having trouble accepting a bottle nipple, with careful observation, you can determine what the problem is. To decide what part of your baby's suck is not working, you need to check the bottle placement in your baby's mouth, the nipple flow and shape, and your baby's reaction to these things, which includes where he places his tongue and lips. The following pictures and explanations detail these specific problems.

Bottle Placement

How you place a bottle nipple in your baby's mouth is just as important as the bottle-nipple choice. In Chapter 5, you learned to wait for your baby to open wide and latch, just as he does with your breast. Next, when your baby latches, it is vital that the nipple is placed deeply into your baby's mouth. Your baby should accept all of the nipple length, as well as a portion of the nipple base. A common mistake parents make is to place only the tip of the nipple into the baby's mouth. This shallow placement may cause the baby to hold the lips in a narrow position and compress with the lips, rather than moving the tongue. The babies pictured in **Figures 8.1** and **8.2** are using appropriate nipple shapes, but here we see a shallow placement.

Figure 8.1

Shallow bottle placement

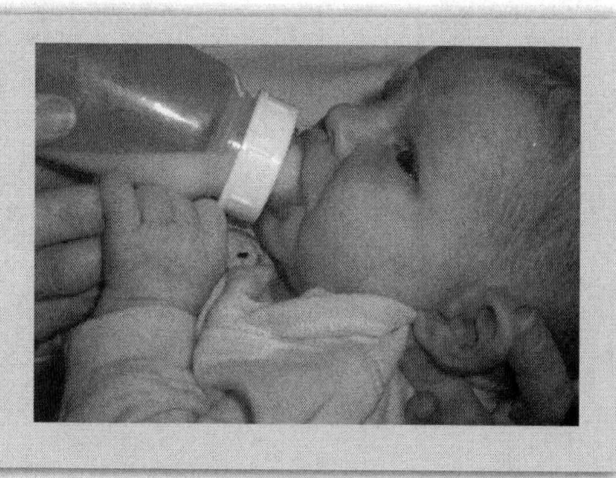

Figure 8.2

Shallow bottle placement

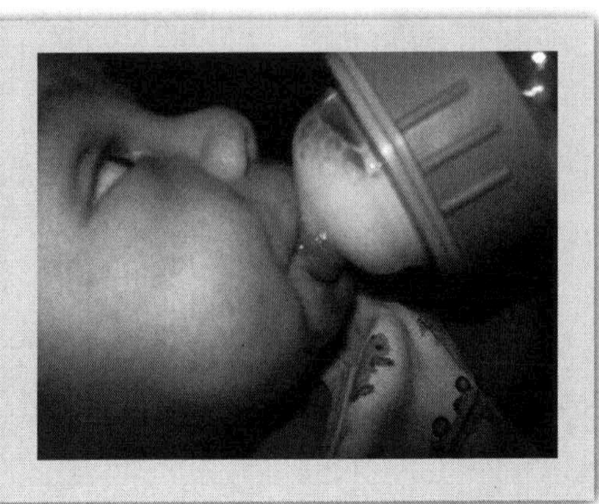

Check Flow

There are two factors that influence the flow rate of bottle nipples. The first factor is the large onset of milk delivered to the baby before the bottle equalizes in pressure. The other factor that influences flow is the amount of milk delivered from the bottle as your baby sucks. Your baby needs to be able to control the amount of milk to create a successful latch. If the nipple is flowing too slowly, the baby may become disinterested, frustrated, or shift from sucking to biting the nipple to extract milk. If the milk is flowing too quickly, the baby may gasp, cry, or choke (**Figure 8.3**). The baby may also pull his tongue back to protect his airway from the large quantity of milk (**Figure 8.4**). When a baby pulls his tongue back, he can no longer suck efficiently.

Figure 8.3

Milk is dripping, baby cannot organize suck and cries

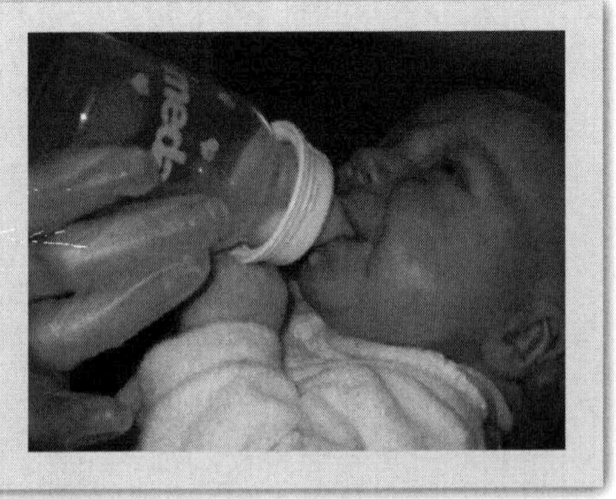

Figure 8.4

Milk is dripping, baby slides tongue to protect airway

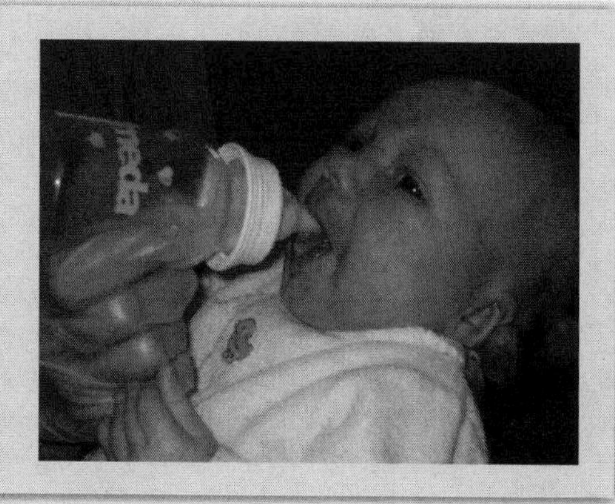

Equalization

You can reduce the large onset of milk at the beginning of a feeding by making sure the pressure in your bottle is equalized. Before introducing the nipple into your baby's mouth, make sure the bottle stops dripping. If your bottle does not equalize in pressure and continually drips, offer it to your baby in an upright position, so the breastmilk is not quite to the tip of the nipple (**Figure 8.5**). Once your baby latches and begins sucking, adjust the angle, so the milk is over the bottle nipple hole (**Figure 8.6**).

Figure 8.5

Same bottle nipple offered to baby, with milk below nipple hole

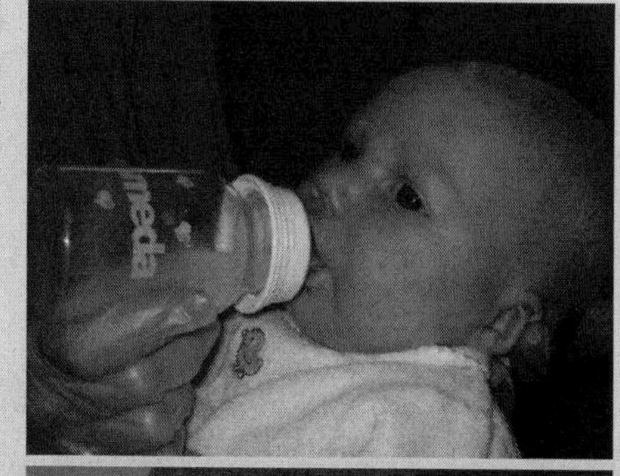

Figure 8.6

Bottle is tipped up, so milk flows after baby's suck is organized

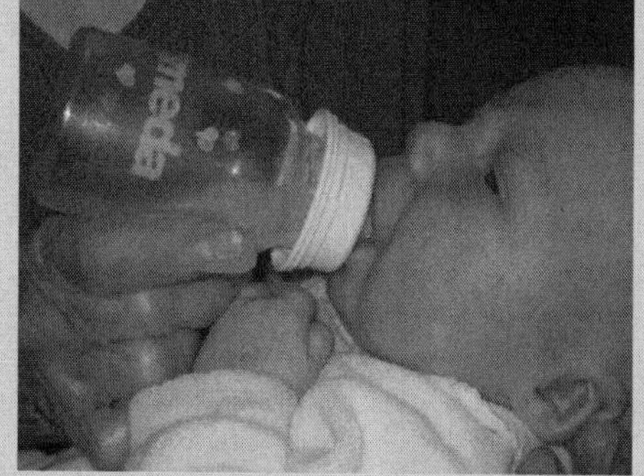

Too Fast

If you notice your baby gulps, looks concerned, or leaks milk from the corners of his mouth, perhaps the nipple is flowing too fast. Feeding in a semi-upright position may reduce the flow. If the baby continues to look worried (**Figure 8.7**), you need to try another bottle nipple, either from the same package or a different brand. A baby who is sucking from a bottle nipple with a correct flow will be calm, happy, and make eye contact with his mother (**Figure 8.8**).

Figure 8.7

Worried baby with furrowed brow, not looking at mother

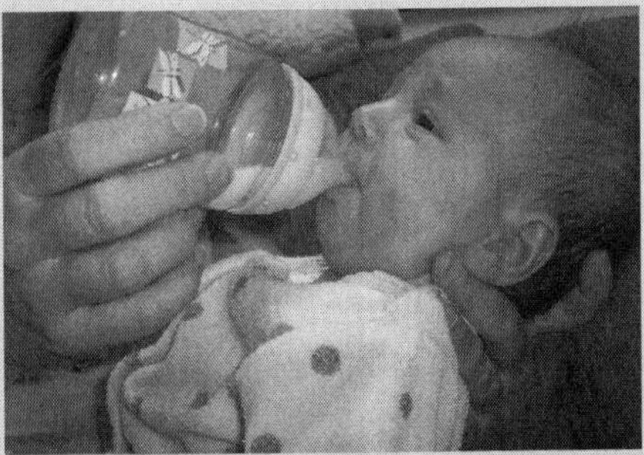

Figure 8.8

Happy baby, good eye contact, calm, easy flow

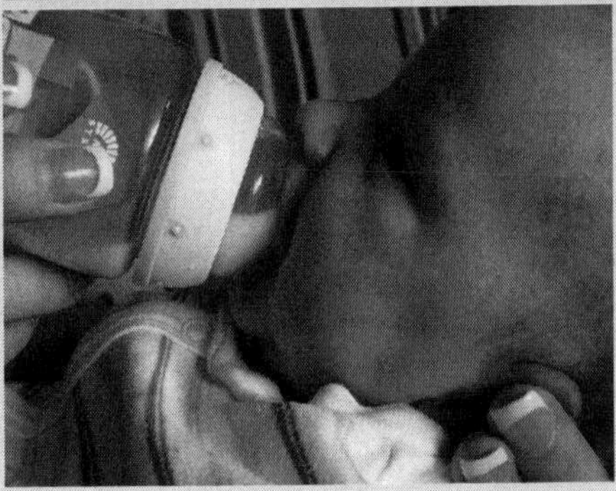

Too Slow

Occasionally, the tip of a bottle nipple may not be completely punched through, causing little or no milk to flow. This is a manufacturing flaw, possibly for one nipple or the entire package. You can suck on the nipple to make sure liquid flows through it. Be sure to wash it before offering it to your baby. If you suspect a flaw, do not punch through the nipple hole. Replace the nipple with another one from the package or try a different brand.

If a bottle nipple flows too slowly, the baby may act frustrated, as though he is working too hard or as if no milk is flowing from the bottle. To compensate for a flow that is too slow, some babies will shift from sucking to biting the nipple to extract milk. The flow of your bottle nipple needs to mimic the flow of your breasts, so your baby does not learn the habit of biting you to extract milk (**Figure 8.9**). A too slow flow, with the baby working too hard, does not protect breastfeeding.

Figure 8.9

Biting the nipple to extract milk, rather than sucking

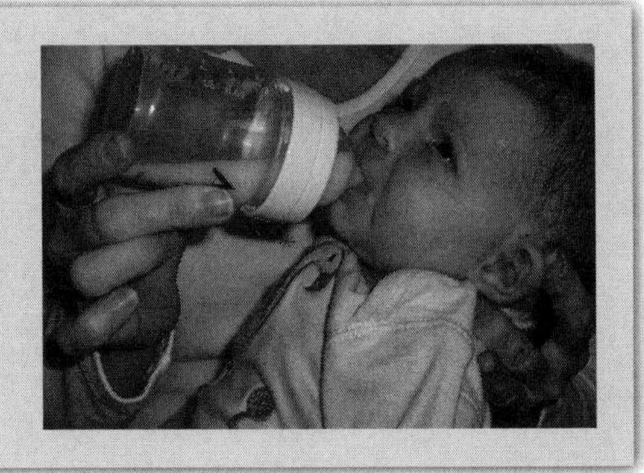

Bottle-Nipple Shape

The shape of a bottle nipple needs to be just right for your baby. Think of the three bears. Your little bear needs his nipple to be "just right," not too short and not too long. There are two length features of a bottle nipple that influence a baby's latch: 1) the overall length of the nipple, and 2) the transition between the nipple length and its base.

The length is important because it should mimic how far your nipple reaches into your baby's mouth. Since the human nipple stretches two to three times its resting length during breastfeeding, your nipple will reach toward the back of your baby's mouth. Artificial nipples do not elongate like the human breast (Nowak et al., 1995). This difference can be controlled in part by choosing a bottle nipple whose length is longer than the resting length of your nipple.

The transition between the nipple length and base should allow for correct nipple placement. Your baby should accept the nipple *and* a portion of the nipple base. Lip placement on the nipple base should mimic your baby's lips on your areola while feeding.

Too Short

When the distance from the nipple tip to the collar is too short, it prevents the nipple from reaching far into the baby's mouth, as a breast does. **Figure 8.10** depicts a baby whose lips touch the bottle collar, preventing the nipple from reaching deeply into his mouth. The nipple shape for this baby caused a host of problems—leaking, tongue moving up and down rather than in a wave, and excessive lip pressure.

Figure 8.10

Nipple too short, lips on collar

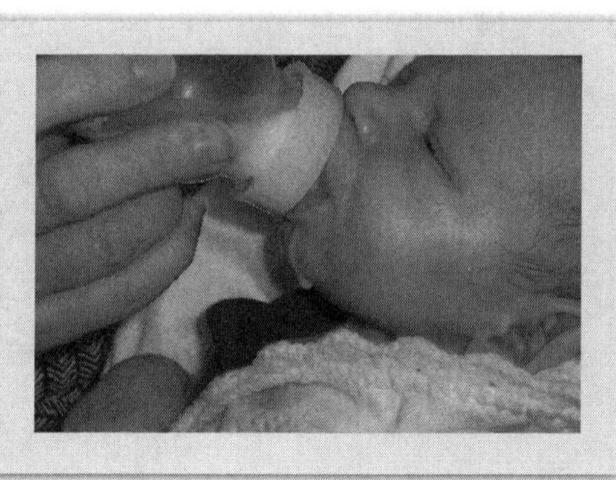

Too Long

When the nipple length is too long, the baby may be unable to accept the nipple and maintain a wide latch on the base without gagging. This shape encourages a baby to suck on the nipple length, promoting closed-mouth feeding. The babies in **Figures 8.11** and **8.12** have accepted the nipple length deeply into their mouths, but have no more room to accept the base.

Figure 8.11

Nipple length too long to accept base

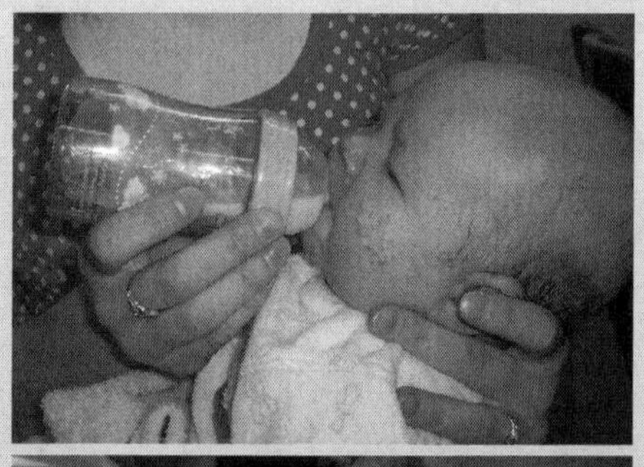

Figure 8.12

Nipple length too long to accept base, causing gagging

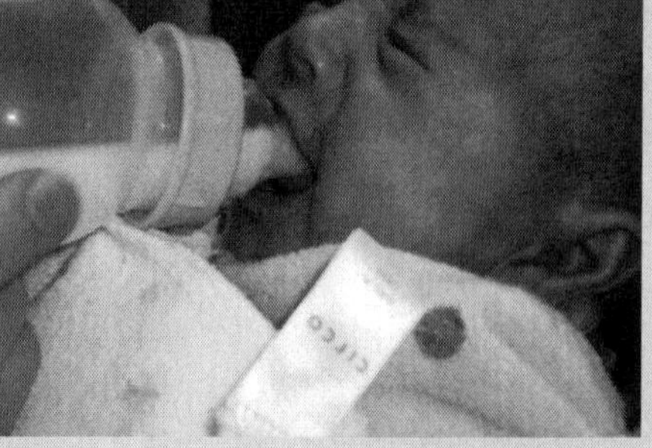

Abrupt Transition

A common misconception is that bottle nipples with a wide base are most like breastfeeding because the mother's breast is "wide." In actuality, many wide nipples have an abrupt transition from base to length, which tends to encourage a baby to feed on the nipple length, without accepting a portion of the nipple base. **Figures 8.13** and **8.14** show gradual and abrupt transitions from length to base.

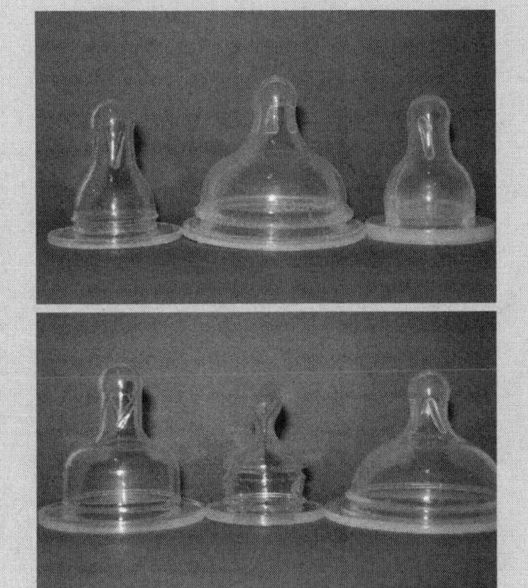

Figure 8.13
Gradual transition from length to base

Figure 8.14
Abrupt transition from length to base

The babies pictured in **Figures 8.15, 8.16,** and **8.17** are using different nipples. They are latched onto just the nipple length, resulting in a closed-mouth feed.

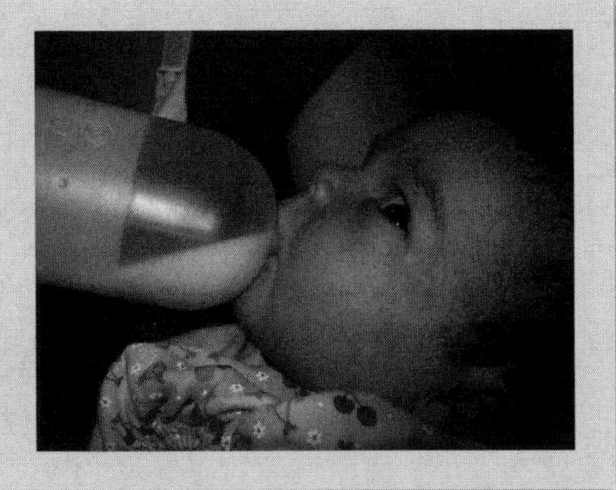

Figure 8.15
Bad latch, averted gaze

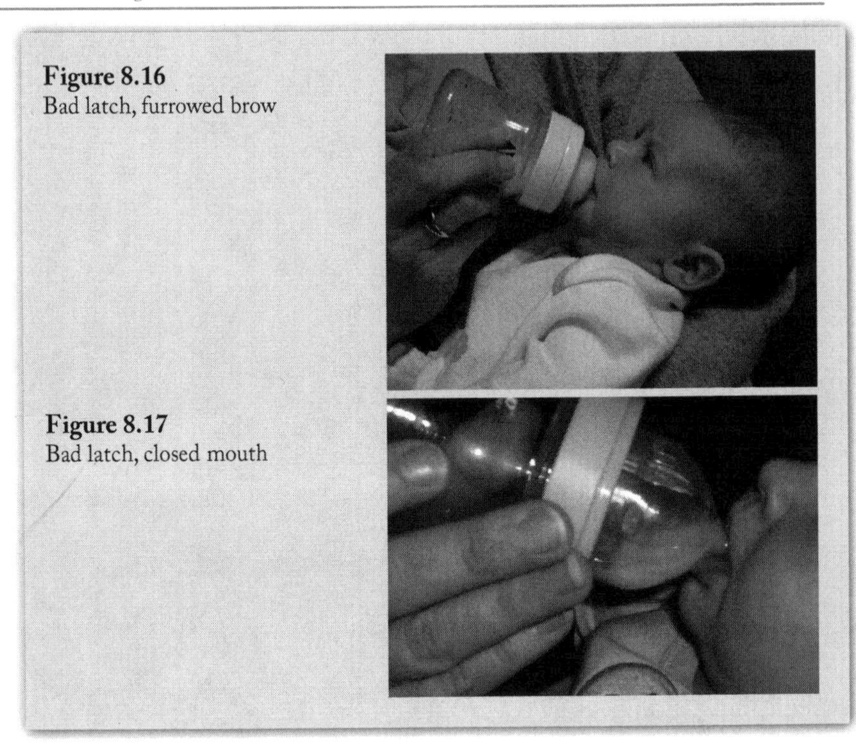

Figure 8.16
Bad latch, furrowed brow

Figure 8.17
Bad latch, closed mouth

If you are trying a wide nipple and your baby does not latch onto the nipple base (**Figure 8.18**), you can create a deeper latch by supporting the bottle nipple in the same fashion you might support your breast to encourage your baby to latch. With your thumb on top of the nipple base near the collar and your fingers on the bottom of the nipple base (**Figure 8.19**), compress the bottle nipple to form a more narrow "bite" for your baby to latch onto (**Figure 8.20**). Once your baby latches, slowly remove your fingers. If your baby can maintain this position, it is a successful placement (**Figure 8.21**). If his lips slip onto the nipple length, try a different shaped nipple.

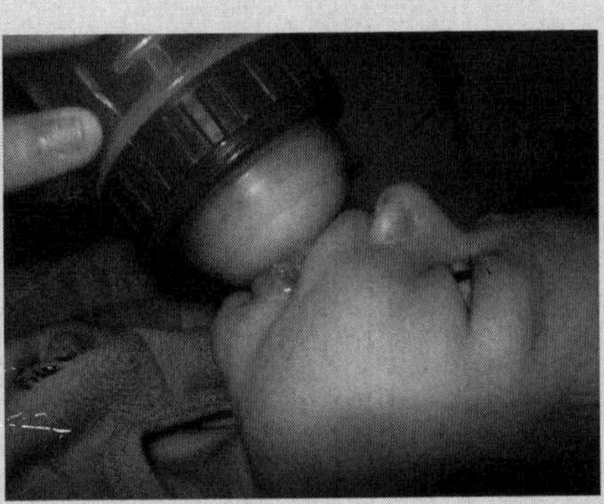

Figure 8.18
Baby's self-led latch is poor

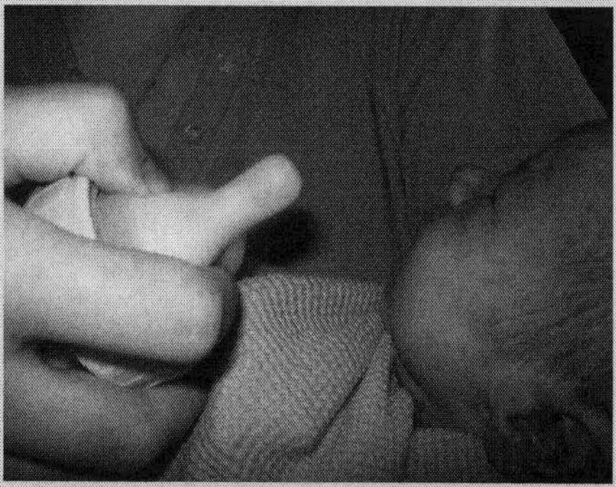

Figure 8.19

Mother compresses nipple base

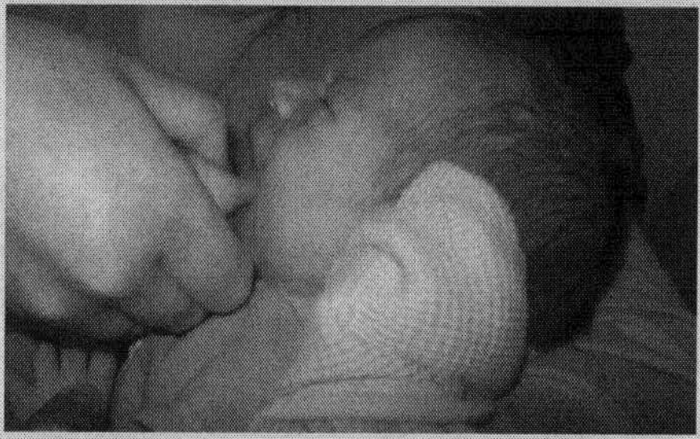

Figure 8.20

Baby opens for latch

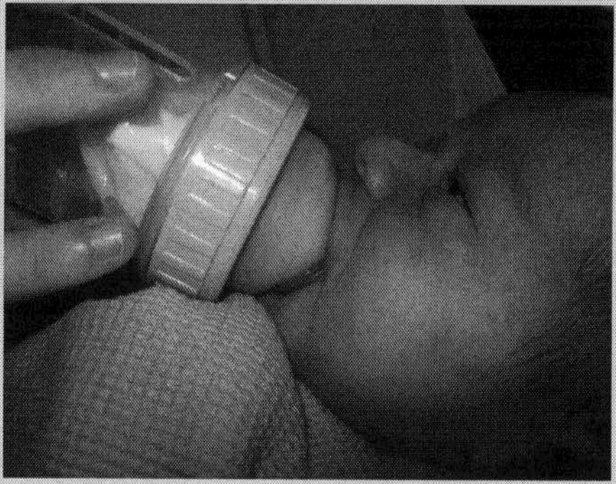

Figure 8.21

Baby's latch is deep

Position of Tongue

Bottle nipples influence tongue position and movement, two important elements of a baby's suck. When a baby does not cup the bottle nipple with his tongue or correctly suck on the bottle nipple, he may bite to get the milk out, not engage his tongue at all, or slide his tongue back and forth under the nipple.

Retracted Tongue

If the nipple shape is a poor choice for your baby, he may pull his tongue back or retract it. Though this can happen with any shape, it is most common with the orthodontic nipple shape. When your baby retracts his tongue, he humps his tongue and bumps the nipple with it. Since his tongue is behind his gum ridge when it is retracted (**Figure 8.22**), the nipple rests on his gums, causing a biting reflex. One study found that one brand of orthodontic-shaped nipples relied on an up-down motion or chewing, rather than negative pressure (suction), like the human breast and other bottle nipple shapes studied (Nowak et al., 1994). This tongue position can be detrimental to switching between breastfeeding and bottle-feeding.

Figure 8.22

Tongue retracted, mouth closed

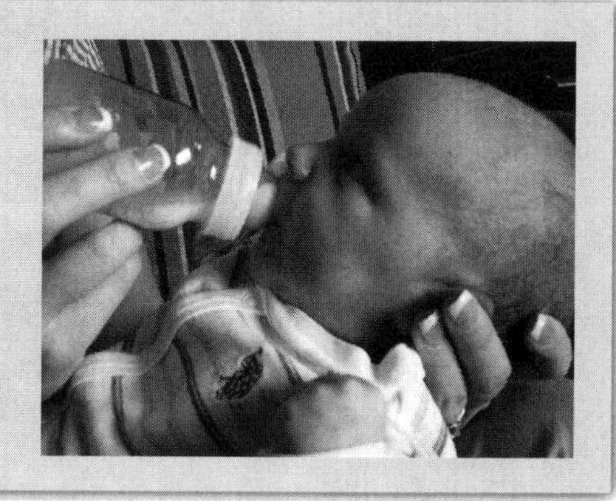

Sliding Tongue

The baby is an active participant in bottle-feeding. He must be willing to accept the nipple and use his tongue for feeding. Sometimes a baby will show his dislike of a bottle nipple shape by not sucking. The baby's tongue in **Figure 8.23** is remaining flat, rather than cupping, and his tongue is sliding back and forth under the nipple. Sliding his tongue causes the nipple to rest in the sides of his mouth. A different-shaped nipple will need to be offered when this happens.

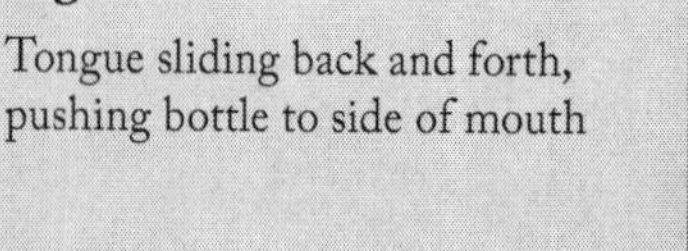

Figure 8.23

Tongue sliding back and forth, pushing bottle to side of mouth

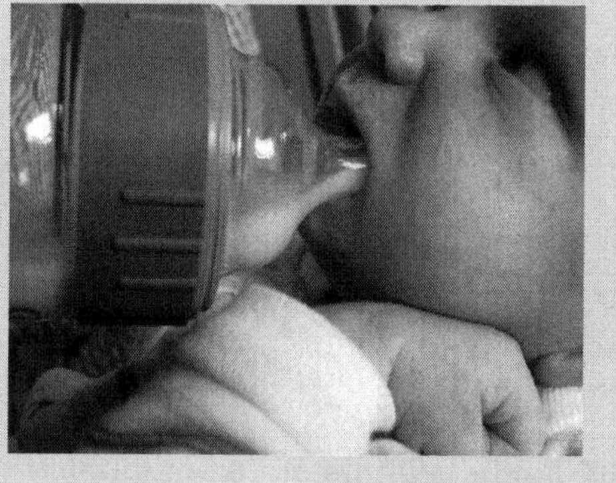

Lips

The position of your baby's lips is just as important on a bottle as on your breasts. Observe your baby breastfeeding. You will notice that his upper lip is visible and his lower lip gently rolls outward, lightly resting on your entire areola. This is the same position and pressure you are aiming for when your baby feeds from a bottle.

There are three common lip placement problems associated with a bottle-nipple latch. Luckily, your baby's lip placement is the most visible component of a baby's suck and easy to assess. First, as stated above, your baby's lips should flip out when using a bottle, not roll under. Secondly, your baby's lips should gently rest on the bottle-nipple base, rather than stretching too tightly. Lastly, the entire top and bottom lip, including the "corners" of the mouth, should be in contact with the bottle.

Flipping the Lip

It is common for a baby's lips to roll *in* when latching onto a bottle, but this is easily corrected (**Figures 8.24 – 8.29**). After the baby latches onto the bottle nipple, use your thumb or finger to roll the lips out. If your baby's lips continue to roll under, the nipple shape may be the problem, and you will need to try a different shape.

Figure 8.24
Top lip rolled in

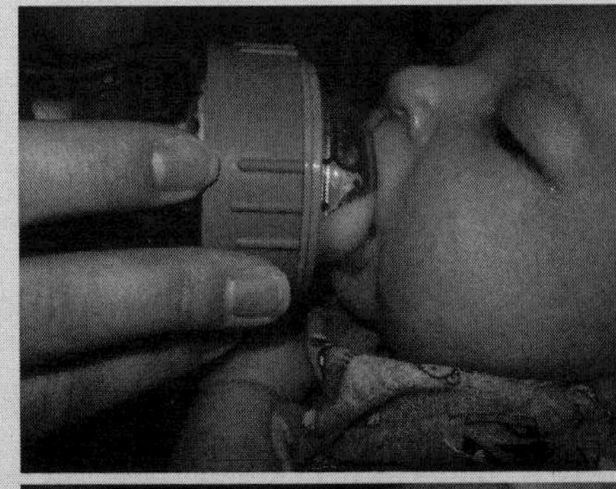

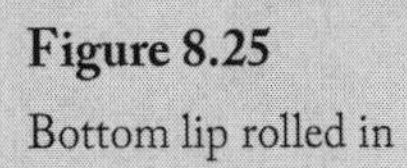

Figure 8.25
Bottom lip rolled in

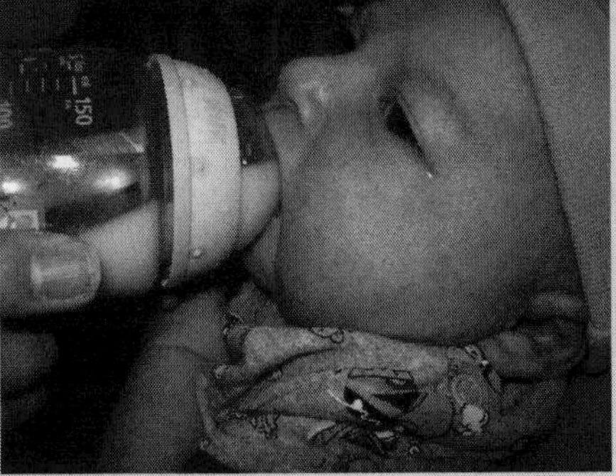

Figure 8.26

Initial latch, both lips rolled in

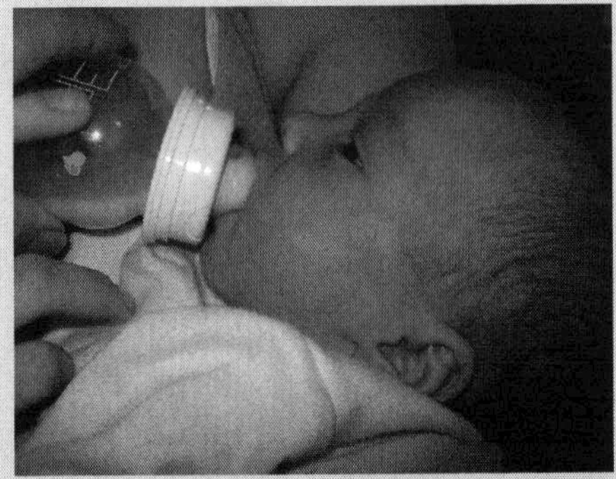

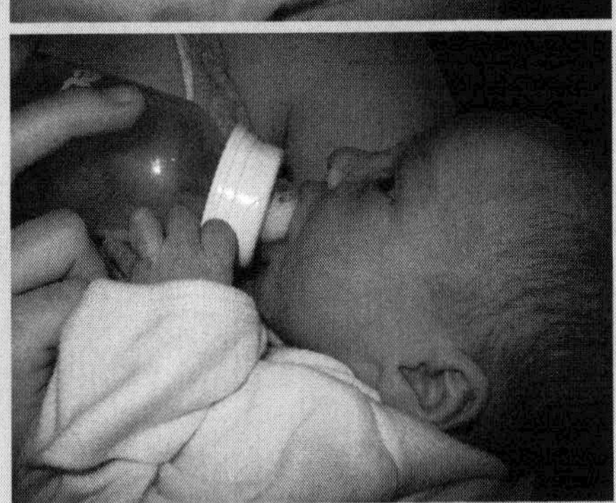

Figure 8.27

Lips flipped out for better latch

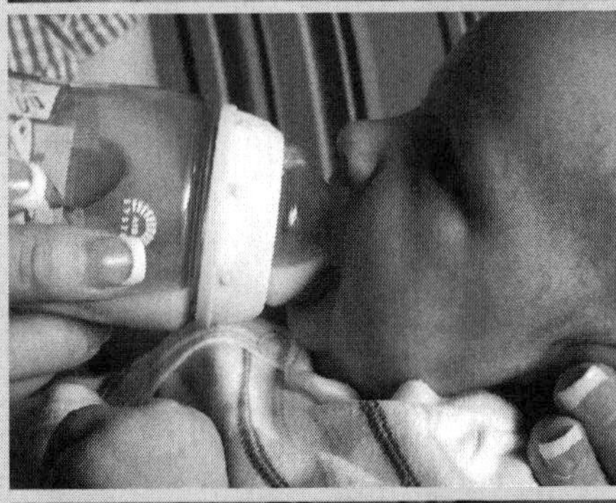

Figure 8.28

Initial latch, top lip rolled in

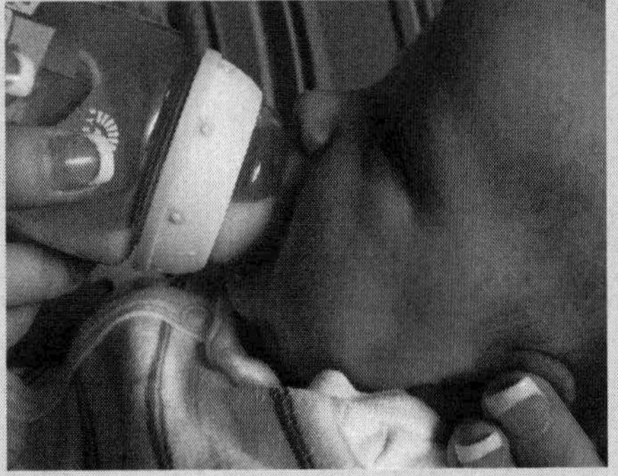

Figure 8.29

Lip flipped out for better latch

Lip Stretched Too Tightly

A baby's top lip should not be stretched abnormally tight. Using a nipple that creates a wider latch than his natural latch on your breast usually pushes and stretches the top lip too tightly (**Figures 8.30** and **8.31**). Try a different shaped nipple if your baby's lip is stretched too tightly.

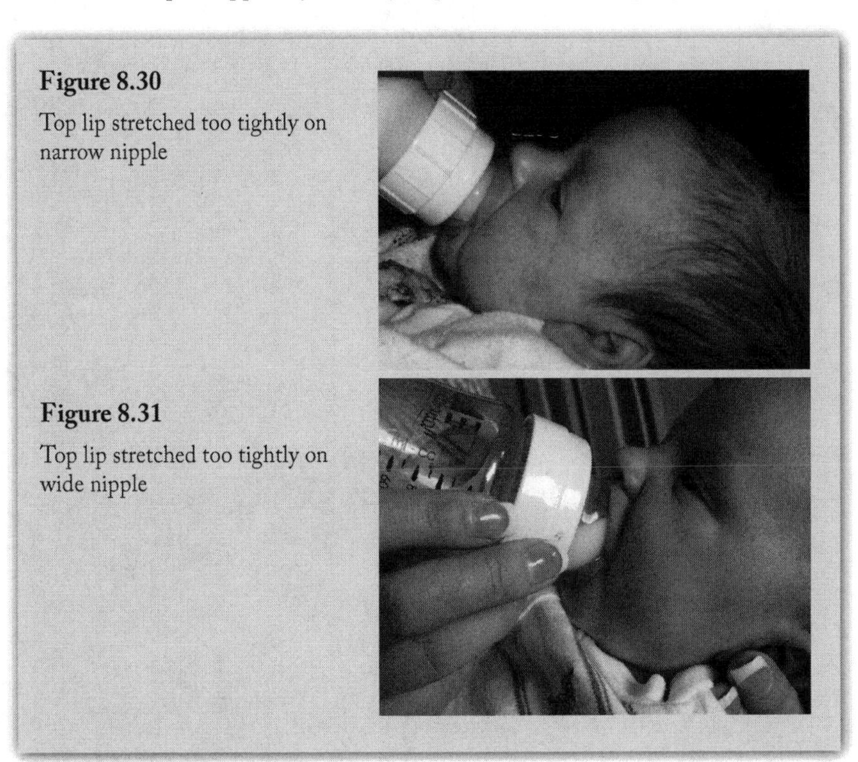

Figure 8.30
Top lip stretched too tightly on narrow nipple

Figure 8.31
Top lip stretched too tightly on wide nipple

Gaps in Corner

Sometimes a baby's lips do not form a seal around the nipple base. This is most noticeable when milk leaks from the baby's mouth. Milk might also bubble in the corner of the baby's mouth. Lack of lip seal can occur when the bottle nipple is too narrow, preventing the mouth from opening wide. Lack of lip seal can also happen when the nipple base is too wide and the baby latches on the nipple length alone, without accepting the nipple base. **Figures 8.32** through **8.34** show poor seals.

Figure 8.32

Too narrow, leaking

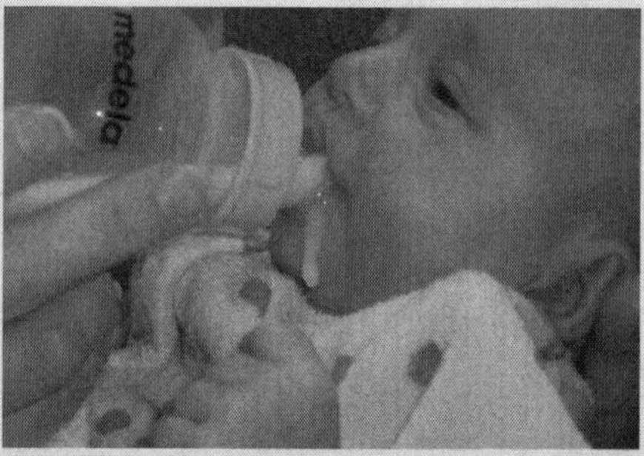

Figure 8.33

Too wide, bubbling at corner of mouth

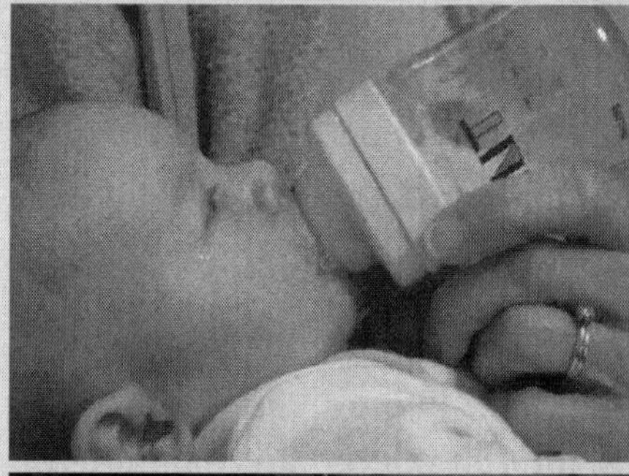

Figure 8.34

Too wide, gap in corner of mouth

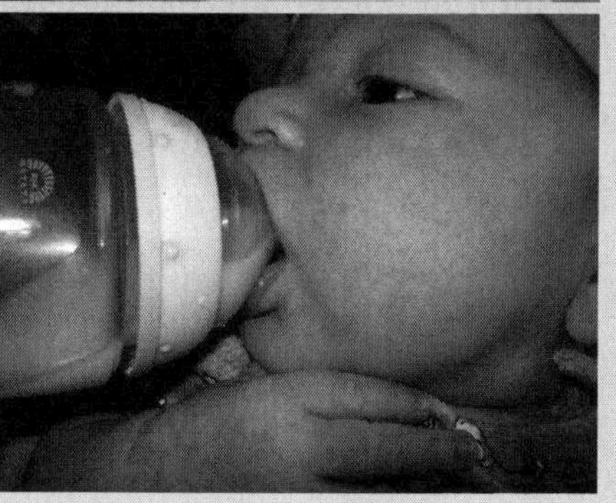

Extra Caution with Certain Nipple Shapes

Orthodontic nipple shapes and nipples with an inner chamber can prohibit the natural flow of milk. When your baby breastfeeds, he swallows 20-30 times with a let-down, then pauses and rests. We have found that these two nipple shapes require the nipple tip to refill, periodically leaving the baby with no milk for his sucking efforts. Nowak and colleagues (1994) found the neck of one brand of orthodontic shape likely to collapse, limiting the amount of milk expressed per suck. We have observed that in order to maintain a steady flow with orthodontic and inner chamber nipple shapes, the baby needs to be held in a very reclined position. This position has been linked to an increase in ear infections (Sears, 2006a).

Crying Babies

Some babies cry when they are learning to take a bottle. What does this mean? There is a difference between a baby who *will not* take a bottle, and a baby who *cannot* take a bottle.

Your baby is "telling" you he will not take the bottle when he closes his mouth, turns his head away, or pushes the bottle away. Try the bottle again by gently touching the bottle nipple to or near your baby's lips. Most babies will latch onto the bottle nipple within a few minutes on their own.

If your baby shows distress by waving his arms about and wiggling, stop and take a break. When you try the nipple later, your baby might benefit from swaddling and the removal of distractions, such as sound and movement (**Figure 8.35**).

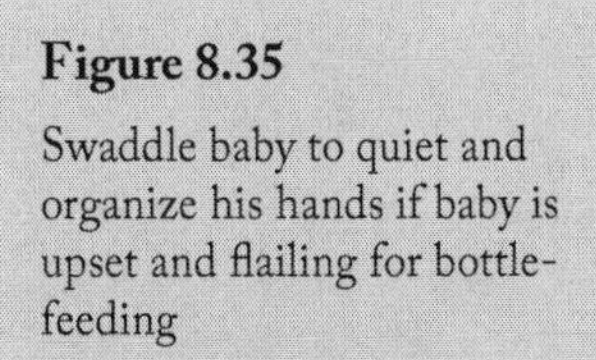

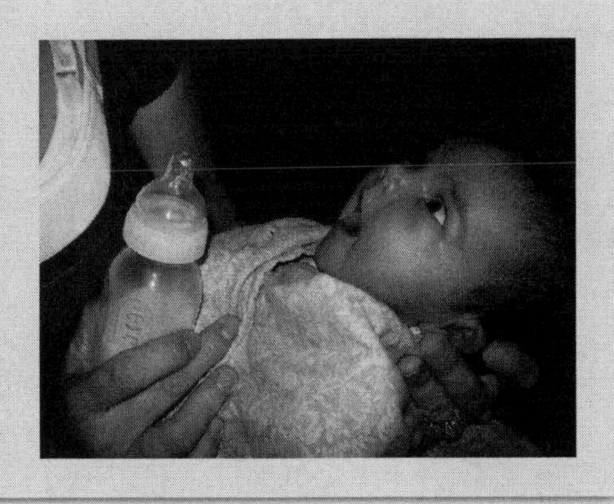

Figure 8.35
Swaddle baby to quiet and organize his hands if baby is upset and flailing for bottle-feeding

If these ideas simply do not work for your baby, try offering the bottle when your baby is just waking up from a nap. Some babies are more willing to try a bottle when they are groggy. If you choose the after-nap-introduction, be sure to offer your baby only a small amount, so the bottle does not replace a full feeding, and then promptly breastfeed your baby to protect your milk supply.

Your baby is "telling" you he cannot suck on the bottle when he tries to take the bottle, but cries instead (**Figure 8.36**). Calm your baby. Try more than one nipple type. The problem might be the shape—does the nipple cause your baby to gag? Use a shorter bottle nipple. The problem might be the flow—does your baby cry as milk drips into his mouth? Invert the bottle for 5-10 seconds to equalize the pressure, or allow your baby to latch in a semi-upright position with the breastmilk not reaching the bottle nipple tip.

Figure 8.36
Sad babies cannot eat

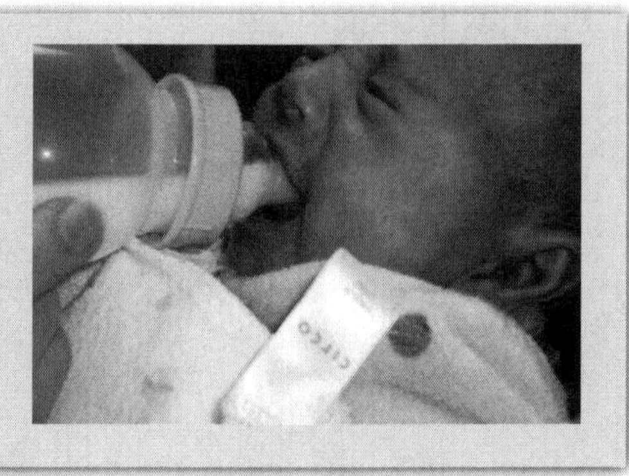

Feedings should not be a sad experience. It is never okay to choose a bottle nipple that drips quickly into a baby's mouth to "make" the baby eat when he will not, or cannot, suck on a bottle nipple. If your baby cries a lot with every nipple you try, stop trying and get help. If you feel your baby *cannot* figure out how to suck on any bottle nipple, we suggest you find a breastfeeding helper to work with you and your baby in person.

Combining Brands

If you have purchased a feeding system and find that your baby cannot achieve a good latch on that specific brand of nipple, you might be able to find a different brand of nipple that works with the bottle you have. Nipples can often be used with another brand of bottle. Many narrow neck nipples can be traded between various brands. Narrow neck nipples work with most breast pump collection bottles as well. Typically, wide neck nipples work only with their own brand, though some nipples and brands are interchangeable.

There are three ways to test if a different brand nipple works with the bottle you have. First, make sure the seam between the collar and nipple base do not leak when you turn the bottle over. Next, the nipple should not collapse (smash flat) when your baby is feeding. Lastly, your baby should be able to pull milk out as he sucks. If one of these tests fails, the nipple will probably work best if you buy the whole feeding system.

Settling

Sometimes it is hard to choose between nipples. Bottle nipples are artificial, and it may be that you are unable to recreate the perfect latch on a bottle. Looking at all the pieces that work together in choosing the best nipple, you may have to "settle" for the closest fit you can find. In **Figures 8.37** and **8.38**, the baby is latched on different nipples. Notice that neither latch is a perfect mimic of a latch on the breast. The explanation of which nipple we chose as "best" for the pictured baby is described below.

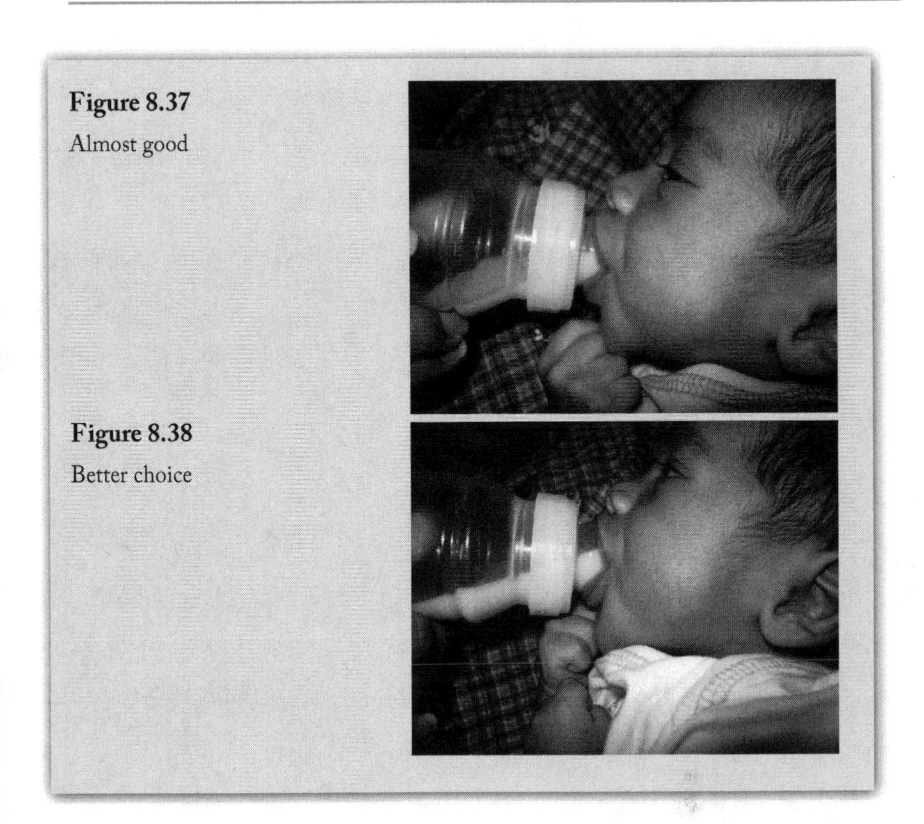

Figure 8.37
Almost good

Figure 8.38
Better choice

The baby is using a narrow neck nipple in both pictures. The nipple on the bottom allows for a slightly wider mouth placement. Also, his suck is more organized, and he is making eye contact with his mother while he eats, a signal that the feeding feels correct to the baby.

A Note About Tongue Tie

Some babies are born with a short lingual frenulum, the membrane that stretches from under the tongue to the floor of the mouth. If this membrane restricts tongue movement, the baby is said to have a tongue tie. We have found that until the frenulum is released by a medical professional, these babies suck more efficiently with a closed mouth position. An abrupt transition nipple with a long nipple length is often the best choice for babies with tongue tie. Once the tongue tie is released, a new nipple can be selected according to the SIMPLE Method.

Chapter 9
Practice Using a Bottle Nipple

Once you have found the best nipple choice for your baby, it is important that you allow your baby to practice feeding with the bottle. There are ways to make these practice times more like breastfeeding. In order to do so, you need to understand the differences between breast and bottle-feeding before you can learn to mimic breastfeeding. However, three differences between breast and bottle-feeding that cannot be copied are length of feedings, change in nipple flow rate, and weaning times.

Practicing

To begin, offer your baby a snack of breastmilk once every day between feedings. It is important that your baby is breastfeeding (at the breast) for his "meals," so your breastfeeding relationship and your milk supply are preserved. Providing ½-1 ounce of expressed breastmilk in a bottle will give just enough milk to allow your baby time to establish the rhythm of feeding with the bottle, but not enough to fill his tummy and delay the next feeding.
When your baby accepts the bottle willingly on a daily basis, you can consider offering the bottle every other day, as long as he continues to take it happily. Practicing once a day, or once every other day, encourages acceptance of bottle-feeding, giving you needed piece-of-mind for when you return to work. If you find he is not happy with the bottle when you move to every other day, go back to daily practice sessions, still as a snack between meals. Some mothers continue to offer a bottle "snack" between each breastfeeding until the baby accepts the bottle happily.

It is common for a breastfed baby who "used to take a bottle" to refuse a bottle all together if he is not allowed to practice frequently. One mother shared with us that her son took a bottle until he was about 3 months old, and then she quit offering it for about 3 weeks. "When I tried to give him a bottle after those 3 weeks, he wanted nothing to do with it." Dr. Karp (2003, p. 178) recommends that parents "not skip more than one or two days...so your baby doesn't forget how to take it." We agree.

When you feel your baby's practice sessions are successful, it is time to teach another adult how to bottle-feed your baby. It is essential to let other caregivers feed your baby, since the goal of bottle-feeding is for the baby to accept the bottle while you are away. Otherwise, if a baby is accustomed to breastfeeding and bottle-feeding *only* with his mother, he might be reluctant to take the bottle from anyone else.

Make Bottle-feeding More Like Breastfeeding

One of the dangers associated with bottle-feeding is that a baby will learn to prefer the bottle over the breast and wean. Identifying the differences between breastfeeding and bottle-feeding is the first step to reducing the risk of early weaning. Controlling the differences is the second step.

There are three substantial differences between breast and bottle-feeding. The first two differences relate to non-nutritive sucking, both at the beginning of a feeding and during a feeding. The third difference is the interaction between the adult and child, or potential lack thereof.

First, the absence of non-nutritive sucking at the beginning of a feeding is a significant difference between breast and bottle-feeding. When a baby breastfeeds, the feeding typically begins with non-nutritive sucking, while the baby stimulates a let-down. The baby sucks for a while before the milk starts flowing. This is different than bottle-feeding. Not only does the milk flow immediately when a baby sucks, but if you have not let the bottle equalize as described in Chapter 6, there is a large quantity of milk that drips out before a baby even latches.

It is important that the bottle nipple is not dripping when it is offered to your baby. Chapter 6 described how to determine if the nipple you are using will equalize in pressure to become a no-drip nipple, and Chapter 8 described how to control the initial flow when your baby starts sucking. Controlling the large onset of milk usually associated with bottle-feeding is one way to make feedings similar to breastfeeding.

The second difference between breast and bottle-feeding is the absence of non-nutritive sucking within a feeding. In Chapter 3, *Understanding Breastfeeding Lingo*, you learned how your breasts have several let-downs during a feeding, which correspond with several intervals of non-nutritive sucking. When your baby breastfeeds, he begins with short, non-nutritive sucks to stimulate a let-down, your breasts provide milk, and as the milk is removed, the flow slows. Your baby pauses and switches to short, non-nutritive sucking again, and your breasts provide another let-down. This happens several times during a feeding.

Not so with the bottle. Once a baby latches and begins sucking, it is possible for the baby to gulp the whole bottle without pausing. This is a significant difference between breast and bottle-feeding. Thankfully, this difference can be controlled.

You can mimic breastfeeding by letting your baby pause and rest periodically while bottle-feeding. There are two ways to pace a feeding. One way is to remove the bottle from your baby's mouth after 20-25 swallows. Allow him to rest for 10-30 seconds, or however long your baby usually rests between let-downs. Then let your baby latch again for 20-25 swallows, and remove the bottle for resting. Repeat this process until the feeding has finished, taking time to burp at least once during the feeding. A similar way to pace a feeding is to leave the bottle in your baby's mouth; after 20-25 sucks, position the bottle so the milk is no longer over the tip. Your baby can rest while the nipple remains in his mouth, as he does with your breast, but the flow will temporarily stop.

Simulating let-downs will help make bottle-feeding more like breastfeeding. This is important in the first few months because some babies who use a bottle may expect the breast to flow in a similar way. Since the breast cannot provide a constant flow, the flow from the bottle needs to be controlled. This technique reduces nipple flow preference.

The third difference between breast and bottle-feeding is the potential for lack of interaction between adult and baby. Bottle-feeding can become an independent feeding method where the baby feeds himself. This can happen with a younger baby when a caregiver props a bottle. An older baby can hold his own bottle and feed himself. You can make a rule that your baby must be in your lap or your caregiver's lap whenever a bottle is used. The interplay between adult and child are important to maintain with bottle-feeding.

When a baby willingly accepts a bottle with ease, it is most natural to offer the bottle in a breastfeeding position, cradled in your or your caregiver's arms. Just like with breastfeeding, making eye contact, touching, and talking with the baby is important. The adult needs to control the flow of the bottle to mimic let-downs. Plan to burp the baby in the middle of the feeding. Switching sides during the feeding is another healthy idea. Continue to hold the older baby during feedings.

Length of a Feeding

On average, we look for babies to finish a bottle in 10 to 15 minutes. It is okay for feeds to take longer when your baby happily feeds, plays while bottle-feeding, or needs extra time for burping. However, if feedings are taking longer than 15-20 minutes *and* your baby seems disinterested or frustrated, perhaps your baby is unable to effectively suck on the bottle nipple he is using. Remember, you should hear swallowing like you hear when he breastfeeds. Either choose a different nipple or go up in nipple size to achieve active swallowing.

Sometimes a baby will slurp down a bottle in less than five minutes. There is a balance between feeds that are too short and too long. Babies need to have enough sucking time to recognize that they are full and to feel calm. A fast feed will leave your baby thinking he needs more, resulting in fussing. Feedings that are too long are also problematic in that your baby may burn more calories than necessary or become frustrated. Make sure you are using nipples with the right flow rate for your baby. If your baby still gulps, try pacing his feedings, as described above.

If you are confident your baby drank enough milk, but a feeding is shorter than 10 minutes, your baby may still act hungry until the milk is digested. Walking, patting, and soothing your baby can distract him while your milk settles. Sometimes a pacifier can be introduced to bridge this time-gap.

Changing Nipple Size/Flow Rate

Mom's flow rate from the breast does not necessarily change as the baby grows, so it is common for mothers to hear that the bottle nipple flow should not change, either. Some breastfed babies will use the size 1/slow flow nipple as long as they drink from a bottle. One mother shared how she fed her baby with the slowest flow nipple. "I found that if she drank from a higher flow, she thought that she didn't need to suck when she nursed! So, we kept her on a newborn slow flow for about 8 months, and then when breastfeeding was down to only a few times a day, she moved to a higher flow."

However, as babies get older, they may need nipples with an increased flow rate. Older babies who breast and bottle-feed know the benefits of nursing: snuggle time with mom, as well as nutritive and non-nutritive sucking. The bottle, on the other hand, is seen as eat, get done, and get down. A nipple that flows too slowly may make the baby feel frustrated. Older bottle-fed babies usually do not want to suck on a bottle for 15 to 20 minutes, although they enjoy breastfeeding for that length of time. Another consideration is that babies tend to eat a smaller amount, but eat more often at the breast, compared with taking a greater quantity less often with the bottle. Again, older babies might object to taking 20 minutes to eat a larger quantity.

It is common for breastfed babies older than 3 months to become disinterested in finishing a bottle if it takes too long, indicating it is time to try a size 2 (medium flow) bottle nipple. If your baby usually eats three ounces in 15 minutes, and starts eating 1½ ounces in 15 minutes and stops, this indicates that the milk no longer flows quickly enough. One mother shared how her 3-month-old was a fast eater, so they went to a faster flow nipple because it made bottle-feeding closer to their normal breastfeeding session. Pay attention to your baby, and choose the best size as your baby grows.

Weaning

Eventually, it is time to wean your baby from a bottle. The American Academy of Pediatrics' book *Birth to Age 5* states, "Most pediatricians recommend that the bottle be given up entirely at around age one and almost certainly by 18 months" (AAP, 1998, p. 279). Introduce a cup around 5 or 6 months, so your baby can begin practicing.

Keep in mind that weaning from the breast and bottle may not happen at the same time. Unlike weaning from the bottle, there is not a suggested timeframe for weaning from the breast. Your baby might begin using a cup during the day when you are separated, but continue breastfeeding at night and other times when you are together.

Chapter 10
Pacifiers

Research says wait to use a pacifier for at least 3-4 weeks (Howard et al., 2003). Why? Let's revisit supply and demand and investigate the potential pitfalls of offering a pacifier. Waiting to introduce a pacifier teaches your body to make the right amount of milk. When your baby sucks on a pacifier instead of breastfeeding, it tells your body to make less milk. Babies who suck on pacifiers often drink less milk, eventually reducing the mother's milk supply. Also, pacifiers require the baby to suck differently than the way he sucks at the breast—to put his tongue or lips in a different position and to move his jaw differently. Many babies cannot remember to change their suck when it is time to breastfeed, and then become "confused."

Say you have waited 3-4 weeks and breastfeeding is going well, as shown by a good milk supply and plenty of wet and poopy baby diapers—is there still a risk to pacifier use? The simple answer is yes, but as you have probably learned, there may not always be a simple answer for your baby. If your baby is happy without a pacifier and you are available to nurse your baby to sleep, great—do not introduce one.

Researchers have shown that pacifier use is related to a higher risk of illnesses, such as diarrhea and ear ache (North et al., 1999). Sexton and Natale (2009) state that prolonged pacifier use can have a negative effect on breastfeeding and can increase ear infections. It has also been proven that pacifier use is positively associated with the frequency of yeast infection/thrush (Mattos-Graner, de Moraes, Rontani, & Birman, 2001). Another negative effect of prolonged pacifier use is early weaning from breastfeeding, though the reason is not understood (Soares et al., 2003). Statistically, babies who *do not use* a pacifier breastfeed longer than babies who *use* a pacifier.

However, do you have a baby who likes to suck a lot and calms and soothes himself this way? If the answer is yes, you may decide your baby needs something to suck on while you are away or if you need a break. Your goal is to have a happy, content baby and to be a happy mom. Choose what works best for you, and minimize the risks of pacifier use by following our guidelines.

Choosing

If you have made the choice to use a pacifier, use it wisely. The first step in doing so is to choose the best pacifier for your baby.

Four popular shapes on the market include orthodontic shape (beveled tip), butterfly shape (flatter, wider shape), cherry shape (bulbous tip), and cylindrical shape. The orthodontic shape (**Figure 10.1**) may cause a baby's tongue to retract rather than cup, so the tongue pushes against the pacifier, and the tongue tip is pulled behind the lower gum ridge, which may encourage biting. The butterfly shape pacifier (**Figure 10.2**) can prevent a baby's tongue from cupping. Because the baby's tongue position and movement are limited with these pacifier shapes, they are not ideal choices for the breastfed baby (Beckman, 2000). A potential drawback of the cherry shape (**Figure 10.3**) is its narrow base, which can encourage a closed mouth position.

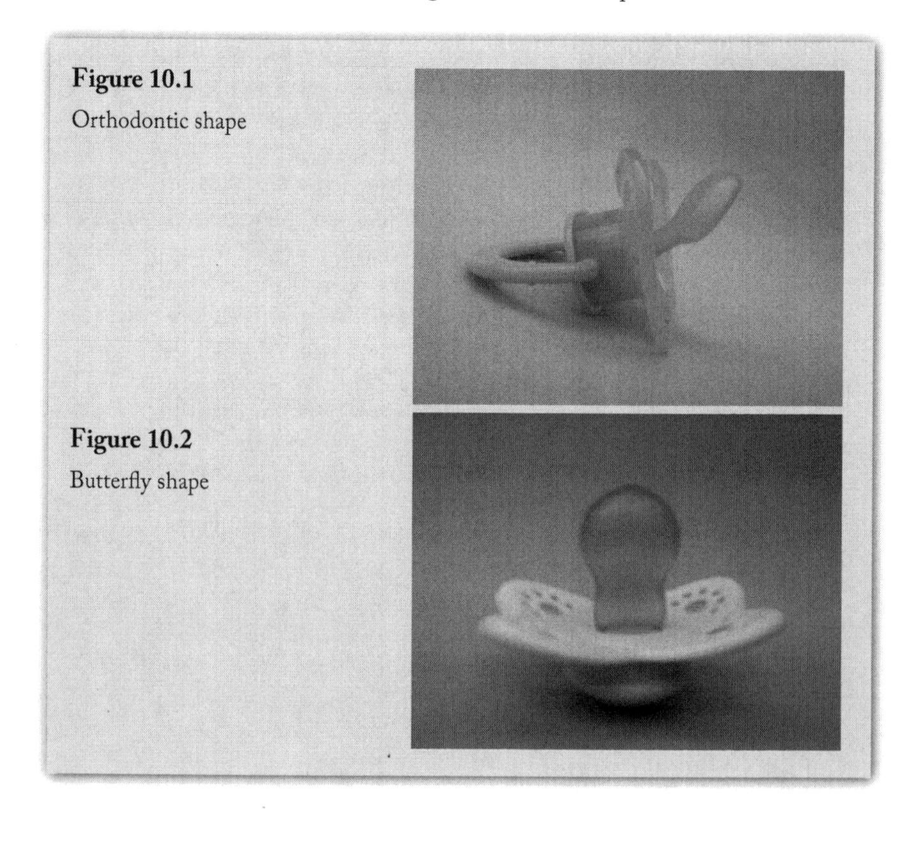

Figure 10.1
Orthodontic shape

Figure 10.2
Butterfly shape

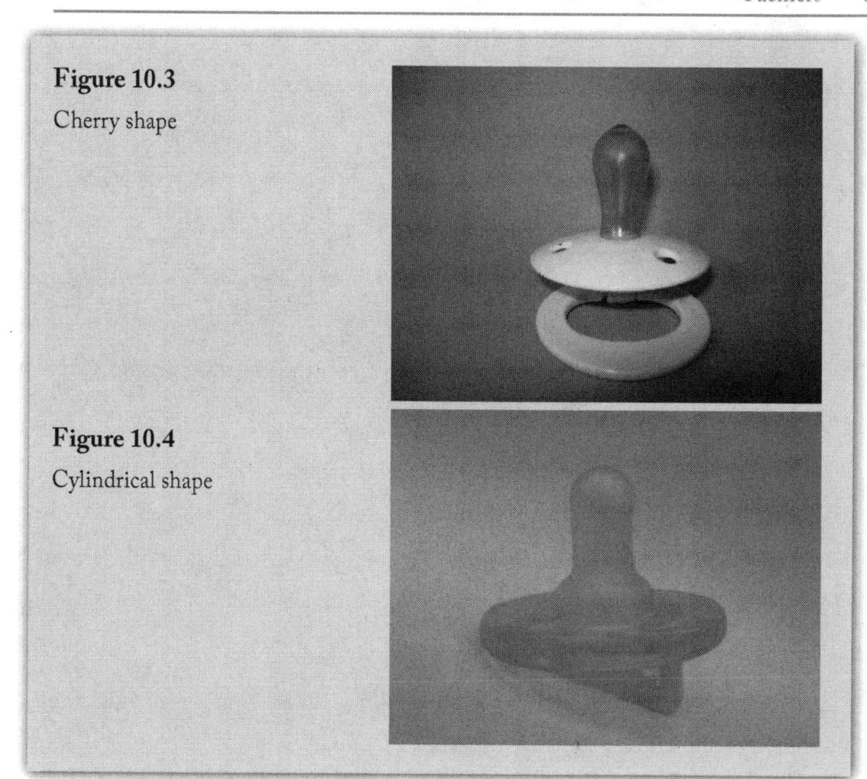

Figure 10.3
Cherry shape

Figure 10.4
Cylindrical shape

The best shape for the breastfed baby is the cylindrical shape (**Figure 10.4**). The cylindrical shape encourages proper tongue placement and movement. When the nipple base narrows (**Figure 10.5**), the mouth is in a more closed sucking position. In some brands, the base of the nipple *slightly* flares (**Figure 10.6**), so a baby's lips retain a slightly wider gape than with other brands.

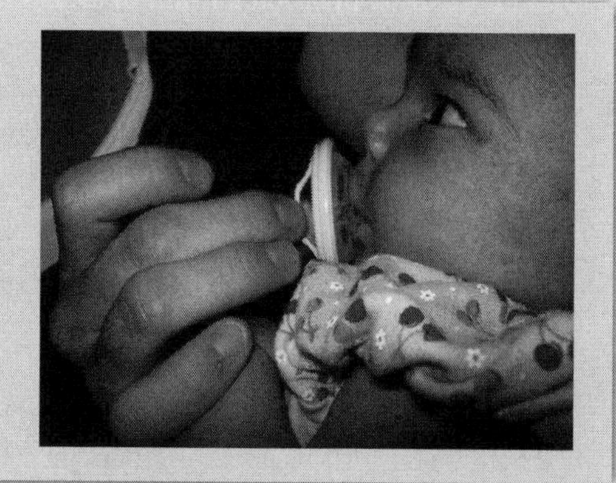

Figure 10.5
Cylindrical style that narrows at base, mouth is in a more closed position

Figure 10.6

Cylindrical style that widens at base, mouth is in a more opened position

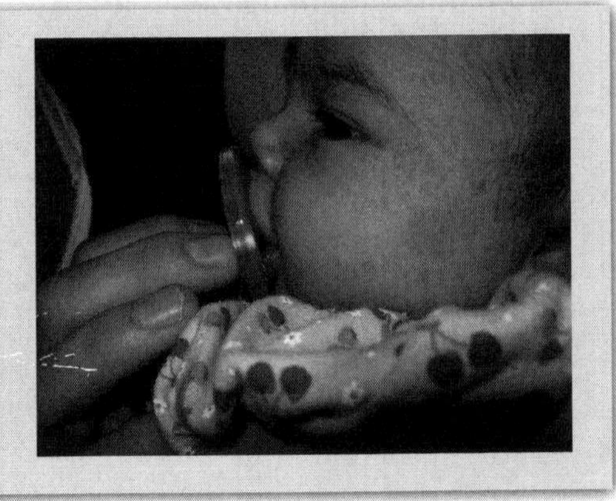

In addition to choosing a pacifier shape, it is important to choose a pacifier for the age of your baby. Newborn (0-3 month) pacifiers are smaller and softer than pacifiers for older babies. Pay attention to the packaging. The right shape nipple may come in various colors, but the pacifier you choose must be for the correct age of your baby.

Some babies either cannot, or will not, keep a pacifier in their mouth. You will know if your baby cannot keep a pacifier in his mouth if it continuously falls out and he cries. If this is the case, your baby may be having issues with his suck, so consider meeting with a breastfeeding helper to learn more (Appendix B). You will know if your baby will not accept a pacifier if he refuses to suck on it or sucks for a few seconds and then pushes it out. Your baby may prefer another shape. For example, if you have a baby who will not take a cherry shape pacifier, he might be successful on a butterfly or orthodontic shape pacifier. With any pacifier, and particularly with these shapes, make sure your baby continues to breastfeed successfully. Stop using the pacifier if breastfeeding changes. Stop using the pacifier if your baby has an increase in illnesses.

Some babies are able to switch between breast and pacifier easily. For these babies, once breastfeeding is mastered, the brand and shape of pacifier may not matter. You are probably wondering if it is best to use the same brand of bottle nipple and pacifier. After reading this chapter, hopefully you will come to the conclusion of "No." Very smart! Currently, the companies that make a pacifier shape which promotes the best tongue position do not make bottle nipples that encourage a wide latch with the same nipple shape. Likewise, the companies that make bottle nipples that promote a wide latch do not make pacifiers that allow for correct tongue or lip placement. If you choose to introduce a pacifier, do not plan to buy the same brand of bottle nipple and pacifier.

If your baby is already using a pacifier, the brand you are using might be okay. If a baby is breastfeeding without problems, gaining weight, and having no difficulties latching onto the breast, the pacifier choice is probably fine. However, if a baby is having trouble latching and staying on the breast during feedings, causing the mother nipple pain, and not gaining weight, the pacifier choice may be a contributing factor.

Using

When you breastfeed or use a bottle, you adjust your baby's lips to flip out and accept a portion of the areola or nipple base. If your baby uses a pacifier that slightly flares at the base, remember to check your baby's lips. Sometimes the lips will roll under (**Figure 10.7**), and they need to be flipped out (**Figure 10.8**). Your baby's suck should be as similar as possible on all nipples.

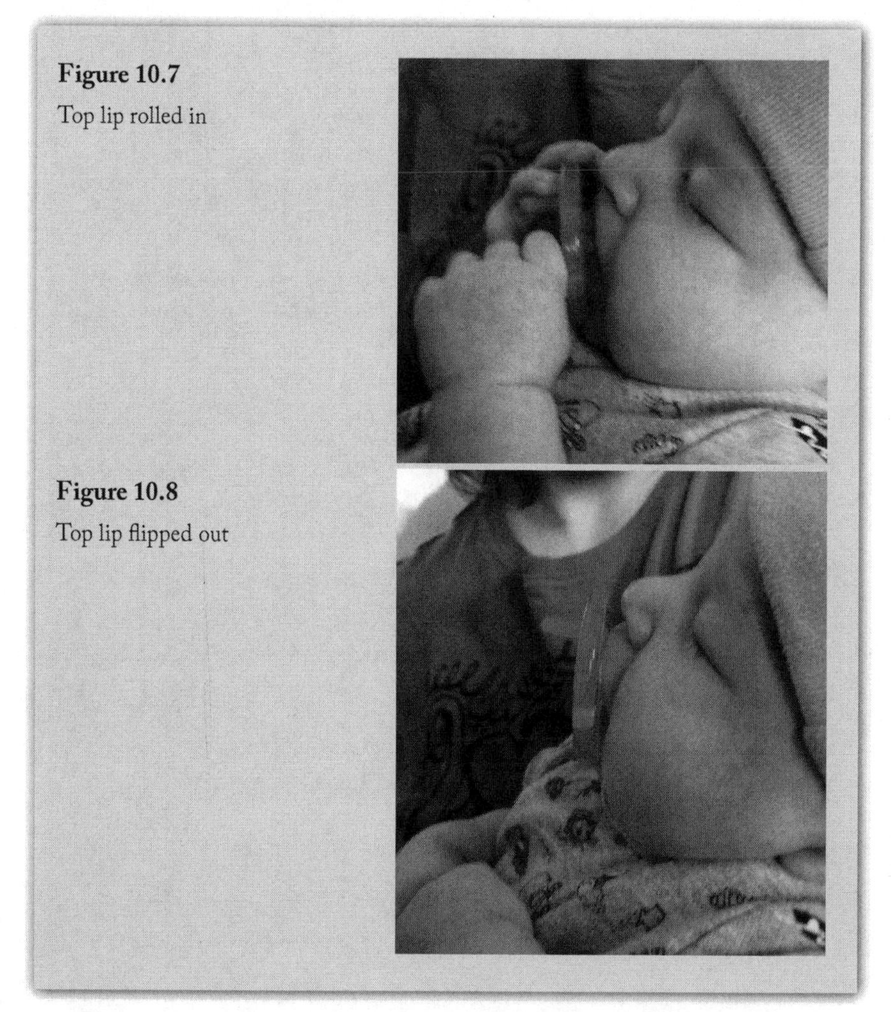

Figure 10.7
Top lip rolled in

Figure 10.8
Top lip flipped out

How often can a baby use a pacifier? Every family's situation is unique. Ideally, save pacifier use for specific times when mom's breast is unavailable, such as when you are separated from your baby, riding in the car, or when you are making dinner. Remember to sterilize your pacifier every day.

To protect breastfeeding, it is important to avoid using the pacifier at certain times:

- Avoid pacifier use 30 minutes to an hour before the next feeding time. If the baby is sucking on a pacifier, he will not be able to show you by his feeding cues that he is ready to breastfeed.
- Do not use a pacifier to space feedings.
- Do not put a pacifier in your baby's mouth because you "think" he is finished breastfeeding. Many babies will breastfeed, digest for 5-10 minutes, and feed again. Using a pacifier breaks this healthy cycle. Also, older babies may become distracted when they breastfeed and want to look around and interact with others instead of eating. Do not mistake this distraction as a sign your baby does not want to eat and insert a pacifier.
- Avoid using the pacifier during a growth spurt.
- Do not offer a pacifier when your baby is content.
- Do not offer a pacifier to satisfy boredom. Instead, change your baby's position or environment.

Too often a pacifier is used to quiet a baby, rather than parents playing detective first. Try to save the pacifier for when you really need it, and avoid using it as a way of life.

If you notice that your baby nurses less often when you are together, becomes fussier, or does not latch on for easy, consistent breastfeeding, do not let your baby use the pacifier anymore. Your baby's breastfeeding relationship is more important than his pacifier relationship.

Weaning

Parents often ask when is the best time to take the baby's pacifier away—the sooner, the better. We suggest it is time to stop using a pacifier in the daytime when your baby is 4 months old. While your baby may feel sad temporarily, young babies are more easily distracted than older babies, so the loss of the pacifier will be an easier adjustment at 4 months of age, rather than waiting. Also around 4 months, many babies are able to grasp toys with their hands. Your baby can now explore toys with his mouth, a necessary part of child development that is sometimes delayed by pacifier use.

Dr. Sears' book, *The Baby Book,* states, "If you have a baby who really needs a pacifier, then use it, don't abuse it, and quickly try to lose it" (Sears &

Sears, 1993, p. 93). In *The Happiest Baby on the Block*, Dr. Karp writes, "Once a baby reaches 4-5 months of age, I usually get rid of pacifiers. By that time, your infant can suck on her own fingers and do many other things to calm herself." He continues, "A baby over 5-6 months may begin to develop an emotional attachment to her [pacifier].... Although you can still wean her from the pacifier after that age, it's often more traumatic" (Karp, 2003, p. 178).

By 4 months, many parents will be equally addicted to the pacifier. Pacifiers entertain babies and make them quiet. Life without a pacifier will involve your time and energy to provide your baby with different toys and environments to explore, and the beginning of speech patterns will emerge (noise!). This is simply part of parenting. Parenting is challenging, and it will be an effort for some parents to give up the pacifier for their baby's benefit. Pacifier use for naptime and bedtime is explored in Chapter 17, *Sleep Like a Baby*. The American Academy of Pediatrics currently recommends that babies suck as they go to sleep, either by breastfeeding or using a pacifier (AAP, 2005). If you use a pacifier to help your baby go to sleep, we still encourage weaning from daytime pacifier use when your baby is 4 months old, and total pacifier weaning at one year.

SECTION 3

Everything You Need to Know About Your Milk

Chapter 11
Storing Your Milk

You work hard to pump your milk. It takes careful preparation and planning to choose the best pump for your situation and to carve out precious time to use it. Make the most of your effort by storing your milk carefully.

How Long

The amount of time human milk can be stored depends on the temperature. Human milk is *best* coming straight from your breast. It makes sense, then, that room temperature would be the next best option, followed by refrigeration, and lastly freezing. Storage time decreases as temperature rises, so buying a thermometer and adjusting your thermostat will allow for the best storage possible. Additionally, temperature is most stable in the *back* of the refrigerator and freezer, away from the door.

Current guidelines for breastmilk storage from the United States Center for Disease Control and Prevention are as follows:

Table 2. Storage Duration of Fresh Human Milk for Use with Healthy Full Term Infants

Location	Temperature	Duration	Comments
Countertop, table	Room temperature (up to 77°F or 25°C)	6–8 hours	Containers should be covered and kept as cool as possible; covering the container with a cool towel may keep milk cooler.
Insulated cooler bag	5-39°F or -15-4°C	24 hours	Keep ice packs in contact with milk containers at all times, limit opening cooler bag.
Refrigerator	39°F or 4°C	5 days	Store milk in the back of the main body of the refrigerator.

Freezer			
Freezer compartment of a refrigerator	5°F or -15°C	2 weeks	Store milk toward the back of the freezer, where temperature is most constant. Milk stored for longer durations in the ranges listed is safe, but some of the lipids in the milk undergo degradation, resulting in lower quality.
Freezer compartment of refrigerator with separate doors	0°F or -18°C	3–6 months	
Chest or upright deep freezer	-4°F or -20°C	6–12 months	
Reference: Academy of Breastfeeding Medicine. (2004). *Clinical Protocol Number #8: Human Milk Storage Information for Home Use for Healthy Full Term Infants.* (PDF - 125K) Princeton Junction, New Jersey: Academy of Breastfeeding Medicine.			

Source:
http://www.cdc.gov/breastfeeding/recommendations/handling_breastmilk.htm
** While current recommendations are five days for storage in the refrigerator, many consider eight days acceptable (La Leche League International, 2008; Biagioli, 2003), though not preferred.

Container Choice

You will need to choose a container to store and freeze your milk. There are many options for milk storage. Expressed breastmilk has the least likelihood of contamination when it is expressed directly into the feeding container. Breast pumps work most effectively when mothers pump into a 4-ounce container. Some mothers purchase several 4-ounce bottles, and use the same container to pump and store their milk. These collection bottles work well with some bottle nipples.

Tully (2000) compared storage containers and found that there is less fat loss with glass and plastic bottles. Additionally, Tully found that the portion of milk that sticks to the walls of the container is more easily redistributed back into the milk with glass and plastic bottles, rather than with breastmilk storage bags. If you have questions about the chemicals in some plastic bottles, such as Bisphenol A (BPA), you can call the product company's toll-free number or visit their website to ask about the chemicals used in specific products.

Despite more fat loss with storage bags, some mothers prefer the convenience. Polyethylene bags designed for freezing breastmilk are the best choice, rather than bottle liners. Some can be connected to the breast pump, so mothers can pump directly into the bags. The fat loss found with bags can be minimized with double bagging (Tully, 2000). If your baby is mostly feeding at the breast, the small amount of fat loss from feeding milk from storage bags is probably insignificant. For a baby who drinks mostly pumped breastmilk, hard bottles might be a better choice. "Rarely would mother's own milk not be the best feeding option, regardless of how it has been stored" (Tully, 2000).

Stockpiling Your Milk

The term "stockpiling" has two meanings. First, as explained in Chapter 4, it means combining the milk from two or more pumping sessions to save for a feeding. For example, if the amount of milk you pump is not enough for a full feeding, you can add the milk to breastmilk you have stored in the refrigerator or freezer. Cool the recently pumped breastmilk in the refrigerator for about 30 minutes, and then add it to your other container.

The second definition of "stockpiling" means to keep a good amount of frozen milk in the freezer for later use. Most mothers who are employed outside the home and will be separated from their babies on a regular basis should consider building up a supply of breastmilk in the freezer. Stockpiling your milk will allow your baby to receive your milk, without supplements, for as long as possible.

The amount you store is determined by your personal goal. You might keep a small reserve "just in case." In *The Milk Memos* by Cate Colburn-Smith and Andrea Serette (2007), the authors suggest keeping a "back up supply of at least three workdays' worth" (p. 29). If your baby eats three 3-ounce bottles at daycare, then storing nine 3-ounce bottles in the freezer meets this goal.

On the other hand, you might be able to store enough milk in the early months, so you can end your pumping career early and still be able to feed your baby breastmilk exclusively when you are apart. One mother who returned to work when her baby was 3 months old, pumped for only 5 months. She built a freezer supply that allowed her baby to receive breastmilk for 17 months! She continued breastfeeding her baby when they were together and sent breastmilk bottles to daycare with her baby when they were apart.

If you decide to stockpile your milk, your baby's feedings will take first priority. There are several ways to pump "extra" milk. Milk supply is highest in the middle of the night and in the morning, when your hormone levels are highest. If possible, take advantage of these times.

- Collect milk from your leaking breast during feedings, using a bottle, bowl, or Milk-Saver.
- Pump in the morning, about 1 hour after your baby breastfeeds. Pump for 10-15 minutes, with the goal of collecting at least one "full" feeding.
- Pump smaller quantities, with short pumping sessions several times a day, and combine the milk.
- Breastfeed the baby on one side and single-pump the other breast at the same time, saving the collected milk.

After you return to work, you can still build a reserve supply by:

- Pumping on the weekend between feedings
- Pumping once in the middle of the night
- Pumping once in the morning, after your baby breastfeeds, but before going to work

If your breasts easily let-down to your breast pump, stockpiling milk may be effortless. If not, pumping and stockpiling may feel overwhelming. In retrospect, one mother shared that she wished she had not felt obsessive about the amount of milk she was able to pump. Her concern about quantity overshadowed the enjoyment of breastfeeding her baby when they were together. Had she to do it all over again, she would choose to live in the moment by enjoying breastfeeding her baby, and not worrying if her baby received some formula when they were apart.

Chapter 12
Using Your Milk

There are many options to consider when filling your baby's bottle. Let's review what we've covered so far. The *Global Strategy for Infant and Young Child Feeding* (the *Strategy*) recommends from the healthiest choice to the least healthy choice:

1. Mother's own fresh milk
2. Mother's thawed, previously frozen milk
3. Pasteurized breastmilk from a donor mother or milk bank
4. Breastmilk substitute (formula)

Recommended length of storage for expressed breastmilk is:

1. Room temperature 6-8 hours
2. Refrigerator 5-8 days
3. Freezer 3-6 months
4. Separate deep freezer 6-12 months or longer

Fresh, Room Temperature

When you will be separated from your baby, providing your baby with fresh, room temperature breastmilk is ideal. Hanna and colleagues (2004) found that antioxidant activity decreased with both refrigeration and freezing. So, mothers who are able to pump once before work should leave a bottle of freshly expressed breastmilk in the diaper bag for the first feeding. Likewise, a mother leaving a baby for a three-hour appointment can express her milk and leave a bottle on the counter for the missed feeding.

Fresh, Refrigerated

Room temperature breastmilk is not always an option, so the next best choice is refrigerated milk, still considered "choice 1" from the *Strategy*. Most of the milk's protective value, like antibodies, is preserved with refrigeration (Williamson & Murti, 1996). Since it is normal for human milk to separate when stored, you may notice layers of fat sticking to the storage container. Fat loss is minimized when the breastmilk is gently swirled prior to feeding the baby.

Since fresh milk is preferred over thawed, previously frozen milk, plan to label and date your milk and store it in the refrigerator if you think your baby might use it (Ezz El Din, Abd El Ghaffar, El Gabry, Fahmi, & Bedair, 2004). If you find your baby does not use it within 5-8 days, add it to your freezer supply.

Frozen

If your baby has not used your refrigerated milk by 5-8 days, it needs to be frozen, considered "choice 2" from the *Strategy*. Labeling your milk with the date of expression and baby's age are recommended. If your baby will be in a childcare setting, label your baby's name as well.

Most mothers returning to work build up a supply of frozen milk. If the milk you are collecting is for your freezer supply, label it and place it directly in the freezer.

It is important to use the milk according to the date of storage (Riordan, 2010). The properties of your milk are specific to your baby's age, so it is ideal to use the milk expressed when your baby is 2 months old when your baby is 2 to 3 months old, rather than 7 months old. Keeping this in mind, remember that your frozen breastmilk, even if it is a few months "older" than your baby, is a healthier choice than formula.

Rotating your stock of breastmilk will help you use the "oldest" milk first. One useful product is the Mother's Milkmate®; it dispenses bottles from oldest to freshest. A simple, gadget-free way to rotate your milk is to use fresh and refrigerated breastmilk through most of the week, thawing 2-4 bottles or bags of frozen milk to use. You can freeze some of your freshly pumped milk to replace the milk you have defrosted. This ensures your milk will be rotated and still allows the majority of your baby's feedings to be fresh milk.

Breastmilk expands when it freezes. Remember to allow an inch or so at the top of the storage container for expansion. If you are freezing into bottles, loosen the cap prior to freezing, and tighten when the milk is frozen. If you are adding fresh milk to already frozen milk, cool the fresh milk in the refrigerator for thirty minutes before pouring it onto the frozen milk to prevent thawing the top layer of frozen milk. If bottle liners are most convenient for your situation, consider "double bagging" to prevent tearing and additional air exposure.

While it is not common, defrosted milk is sometimes described as having a soapy smell. This can occur when milk is stored in a self-defrosting freezer and is caused by changes in the milk fats. This milk is safe to use, and babies are still willing to eat this milk when this happens.

Another uncommon problem is when milk turns rancid after storage. Some mothers produce milk high in lipase, an enzyme that breaks down fat (Mohrbacher & Stock, 2003). When milk high in lipase is refrigerated and/or frozen, it becomes rancid. Babies refuse to feed when this happens. If you will be storing milk regularly, we suggest you test your milk. Heating milk that is already rancid will not reverse this change, so take time to test your milk (Tully, 2000).

You can perform a simple "smell test" to rule out this problem. Express some milk. Store some of the milk in the refrigerator and the rest in the freezer. In one week, defrost your milk. Smell both the refrigerated container and the frozen container. If it has a rancid odor, you will need to treat your milk before storing it.

If your milk is high in lipase, you can inactivate the lipase by scalding your milk before storing it (Lawrence & Lawrence, 1999). Express your milk. Pour it into a pan and scald the milk. Scald means to heat the milk until it is bubbling on the sides of the pan, but *not* a full boil. Remove it from the heat, and quickly cool your milk in the refrigerator or freezer for storage.

Donor Milk

The third choice for baby milk is donor milk. Donor milk typically comes from human milk banks, with the recipients being premature babies and children with specific healthcare needs. Human milk banks have strict screening procedures, including blood testing. They pasteurize breastmilk, so it is safe to give to another, non-biological child. It is not recommended that mothers casually share extra breastmilk due to inherent health risks. This information may sound familiar because it is the same rationale as to why borrowing or sharing a breast pump is not recommended. Perhaps someday milk banks will be well stocked and able to supply every interested mother and baby with additional breastmilk. Until then, stockpiling your milk is the best option.

Breastmilk Substitute (Formula)

The last choice of baby milk is *formula*. Even so, some mothers employed outside the home will eventually combine breastfeeding with formula feeding. The longer your baby is able to receive your milk alone, the better. If you do need, or choose, to add formula to your baby's diet at some point, try to maintain some breastfeeding for as long as possible. *Some* breastfeeding is a healthier choice than *no* breastfeeding.

Warming

When you are ready to feed your milk to your baby, you may notice your milk has separated into several layers. This is normal. Gently swirl your milk to combine the layers, and to redeposit fat that may have adhered to the sides of the storage container. Never shake your breastmilk because it can damage the molecular shape of the protective proteins, an important part of your milk (Smith, 1998). Some babies will happily drink cold breastmilk. If your baby prefers warm milk, be careful not to overheat your milk, as this can destroy lipase, a part of your milk that helps your baby digest fat (Tully, 2000). There are several ways to defrost and warm milk. You may defrost your milk in the refrigerator, which can take 12 hours. Another method is to run cool water over the container, gradually increasing the heat to warm as it defrosts. Another way to defrost milk is to fill a large cup or pitcher with warm water and place the sealed bottle in the container for several minutes. If the milk is in a bottle liner and the water becomes cloudy as the milk defrosts, this indicates a hole in the storage bag, and it is recommended that the milk be discarded. There are products on the market to aid in defrosting, such as bottle warmers. It is not recommended to let frozen milk defrost at room temperature. Do not microwave human milk or warm it on the stove.

Chapter 13
Your Milk Supply

For most mothers, the amount of milk produced is based on supply and demand. When milk is removed from your breasts, your body receives the signal to make more. When your breasts become overly full for an extended period of time, your body receives the signal to slow production. Pumping at frequent intervals can help you avoid the slowing of production. Despite frequent pumping during separation, your milk supply may drop. We have listed below many tricks for maintaining and boosting your supply.

Maintaining Your Supply

It is important to remove the milk from your breasts often when you are working or separated from your baby. Your baby will thrive because he will have your milk when you are apart, and your body will remember to keep making milk because you are pumping. There are numerous ideas to keep your supply plentiful.

- Breastfeed often and avoid using the bottle or pacifier when you are with your baby.
- Try to pump at least every three hours when you are separated.
- Use a high quality, double electric breast pump as described in Chapter 4, *Choosing and Using a Breast Pump.* The right pump is key. It helps maintain supply. If you have been using a less-than-best choice, switching to a higher quality pump may help turn your supply around.
- Rebuild your milk supply on weekends. Breastfeed your baby as often as he is willing; a baby's suck is more effective than a breast pump.
- Ask your baby's caregiver not to feed your baby within an hour of your return. If your baby cannot wait, limit the quantity to 1 ounce or less. Breastfeed your baby at daycare before taking your baby home.
- Keep in mind that certain medications, such as decongestants, cold medicines, and birth control, can reduce your milk supply.
- Drink to thirst and eat a well-balanced diet. Drinking too much water can decrease your milk supply. Choose some drinks with calories.

Boosting Your Supply

Mothers who return to work sometimes find it challenging to maintain a full milk supply. It is normal for your milk supply to be highest on Monday and to decrease by Friday. If your supply is not meeting your baby's needs, here are some tried-and-true ways mothers use to maintain their milk supply.

- Pump in the middle of the night when your hormone levels and milk supply are highest.
- Try pumping one breast while the baby breastfeeds on the other side.
- Double pump after breastfeeding to signal your body to make more. This is like simulating a growth spurt.
- Try to add an extra pumping session at the workplace.
- Apply heat to the breasts prior to pumping.
- Gently massage your breasts during pumping.
- Continue pumping for two minutes longer when your breasts stop dripping milk. Do not turn the vacuum higher. This will not boost your milk supply and will make your nipples sore.
- Let the nonessential tasks go for a few days, devoting more time to breastfeeding, resting, and reducing stress.
- Discuss herbal or medicinal options for boosting your milk supply with your healthcare provider.
- Take an afternoon off to rest and breastfeed frequently.

Providing your baby with your breastmilk while you are separated is a big commitment. Mothers who make this choice can feel proud of their efforts. One mother shared that "it was tough at times," but for her baby, it was worth it.

Persistent Low Supply

When babies breastfeed effectively and often, most mothers will usually have a plentiful milk supply. For mothers who consistently have low supply problems, please read *The Breastfeeding Mother's Guide to Making More Milk* by Diana West and Lisa Marasco (2009). This book is solely devoted to identifying and overcoming milk supply issues.

SECTION 4
Putting it Together

Chapter 14
Your Workday

Providing milk for your baby influences your daily routine. Your routine will now need to include selecting an outfit for pumping ease and packing the pumping supplies you will need while away from home (Appendix D). A planned morning is essential to allow for communication between you and your baby's care provider before leaving your baby. Once at work, you will need to pump your milk to keep up your supply and provide your baby with your milk. Not all work places are ideal for pumping at regular intervals. We have included a table of options to help you select the best pumping schedule for you, and time saving tips for cleaning your breast pump (**Table 3**).

At Home

Ideally, plan to begin the day with breastfeeding. If you are lucky, you can breastfeed your baby back to sleep, and then have time to get ready without your baby in arms. If your morning is going well, try to squeeze a pumping session in, as your milk supply is high. Send this bottle in the diaper bag for your baby's first meal while you are apart.

When you get dressed in the morning, choose a two-piece outfit with easy access to your breasts. Your breasts will be larger than before your pregnancy. Try your blouses on a week or two before returning to work, so you have time to adjust your wardrobe if needed. Since leaking milk may be an issue, choosing an easy-wash fabric with a print is ideal. Consider adding layers, such as a light jacket, which you can slip on in case you leak.

Leaking breasts are often a side effect of breastfeeding. There are four ways to lessen this potential embarrassment. First, expressing regularly can reduce leaking. Next, if you feel a let-down coming, discreetly apply pressure to your nipples, such as folding your arms across your breasts, to prevent leaking. Another defense is to wear nursing pads, keeping in mind to change them at each pumping interval to reduce the possibility of thrush, a yeast infection. Lastly, consider using a product like LilyPadz®, a silicone shield that applies pressure on the nipples to prevent leaking.

Most mothers purchase a few nursing bras that make breastfeeding and pumping more convenient. Some nursing bras have special slots to secure the breast pump flange. Some bras and pumps have attachments, so you are able to pump "hands-free." Another option that works with any bra and pump is the Easy Expression™ Bustier (**Figure 14.1**). It is like a tube top that zips in the front, easy to put on just before pumping. It holds the flanges securely in place, so you are able to continue working or take a few minutes to yourself while you pump.

Figure 14.1

Hands free pumping with Easy Expression™ Bustier

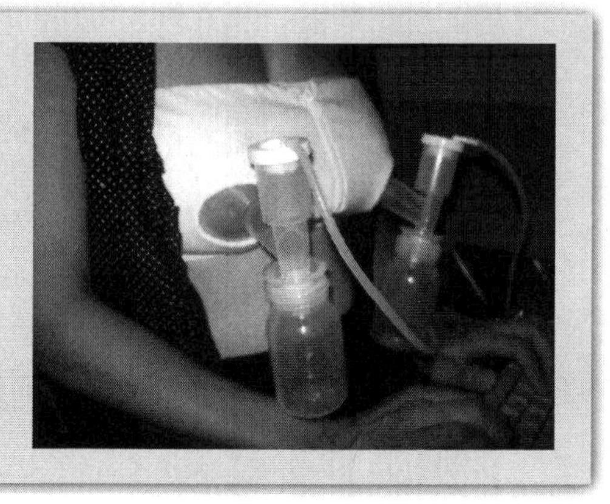

When you pack a bag for your baby, remember to pack your bag, too. The items for your bag (below) are also listed in Appendix D.

- Breast pump with all parts and tubing
- Extra filters/membranes: one set attached to your breast pump, an extra set stored in your bag
- Two 4-ounce bottles or collection bags for each pumping session
- Power supply: extension cord, extra batteries
- Ice packs and tote, or refrigerator container
- Cleaning method of choice
- Nursing pads if your breasts leak
- Baby mementos: picture, blanket
- Easy Expression™ Bustier optional
- Nursing CD/MP3

Dropping Your Baby Off

Leaving your baby is an emotional event. Pack some tissues and wear waterproof makeup. On the happy side, breathe a sigh of relief that you have helped your baby learn to bottle-feed. Your baby is one of the lucky ones who will eat when his mother is at work. One mother shared with us how relieved she felt that bottle-feeding was an easy transition because there were other unanticipated transitions at daycare, such as naptime and simply being separated for a longer stretch of time.

It is important to take time to communicate with your childcare provider about your baby's feedings on a regular basis. Your childcare provider needs to know your preferences regarding storage, quantity of feeds, warming, refrigerating or reusing milk, and the end-of-the-day bottle. This is explored further in Chapter 15, *Your Baby's Day*.

Pumping Scenarios

How does pumping transfer to the work place? The answer will be different for every mother. Your type of employment can dictate how often you can pump.

In a perfect world, a mother has on-site childcare and can breastfeed her baby, rather than pump. This is not an option for most moms, though. The next best choice is to pump at regular intervals—as often as your baby would breastfeed, or at least every three hours. Applied, this often means a morning and afternoon pumping break, in addition to pumping over lunch. Even this is not realistic in all situations.

The availability to pump at work will often make or break the breastfeeding relationship—but it does not need to. One mother shared with us how she worked outside the home fulltime, and since she did not have time to pump at work, her milk supply was waning. If you share this mother's situation and find you cannot pump at work, you still have options. Since your milk supply is highest during the night and morning hours, consider taking advantage of your increase in supply and pump. Some mothers can pump once at night and have enough milk for their baby the following day. Adding a pumping session before leaving for work often yields a high quantity as well.

If you find your breasts do not cooperate with an abundance of extra milk for these pumping sessions, take heart. Any breastmilk your baby receives is healthier than no breastmilk. Even if your baby receives some formula during your absence, you can continue to breastfeed when you are together. It is okay to supplement and keep breastfeeding. Your body learns when to make milk. If you breastfeed your baby every morning, evening, and during the night, your body will maintain milk production during these times, even if you do not pump during the day. On your days off, you will likely need to follow a similar schedule of supplementation during your normal work hours coupled with breastfeeding, but pay attention to your body to determine the best balance for you. Breastfeeding is more than nutrition; it lays the foundation for good health, attachment, and numerous other benefits. You can still breastfeed your baby, even if you cannot pump at work.

Table 3 gives some ideas you can adjust for your own situation. Remember to add time for clean-up.

Table 3. Ideas for Pumping at Work, Beginning with the Ideal Scenario

	Morning Break	Lunch Break	Afternoon Break
Scenario 1 (ideal)	Onsite daycare: visit baby and breastfeed	Onsite daycare: visit baby and breastfeed	Onsite daycare: visit baby and breastfeed
Scenario 2	Pump 10 minutes	Visit baby and breastfeed	Pump 10 minutes
Scenario 3	Pump 10 minutes	Pump 10-20 minutes	Pump 10 minutes
Scenario 4	Pump 5 minutes to relieve engorgement and prevent leaking	Pump 10-20 minutes	Pump 5 minutes to relieve engorgement and prevent leaking
Scenario 5		Deduct 15 minutes from your lunch break to create one morning or afternoon break: "created" breaks pump 10 minutes, lunch break pump 10-15 minutes	
Scenario 6		If your lunch break is not long enough to divide into a separate pumping break, come to work 10 minutes earlier or stay 10 minutes later to accommodate one extra pumping session: "created" break pump 10 minutes, lunch break pump 10-15 minutes	
Scenario 7		Pump 10-20 minutes	
Scenario 8	Pump to relieve engorgement until your supply diminishes during hours of employment, but continue to breastfeed your baby when you are together.		

Cleaning Up

When making a plan, consider how long you wish to pump and calculate additional time for refrigerating milk and clean up. Manufacturers recommend washing pump pieces (flanges, filters, bottles) with warm soapy water after each use. Pieces need to be dried before storage or left to air dry on a drying rack or clean towel.

If you do not have access to a sink or privacy, or when time is limited, there are other ideas to consider. First, some mothers buy an extra set of flanges and bottles, so they have additional collection parts to use while at work, cleaning everything later at home. Another idea is to use wipes made for cleaning breast pump parts. If a sink is not available, several companies make sanitizing wipes specifically designed for cleaning breast pump pieces; no water is required. When using sanitizing wipes, it is recommended that pump pieces air dry for 10 minutes before subsequent use or be rinsed with water. If you have time to wash your pump pieces at work, you can save drying time, or shelf-space needed for drying your pump parts, by keeping them in a mesh bag and hanging them to air-dry at your desk or with your other belongings. Being creative with your choice of clean-up methods allows for more time to be spent pumping.

Another time saving technique is refrigeration. Instead of cleaning pump pieces after each use, one mother shared that she kept her pump parts pre-assembled and placed them in a zipper-top gallon storage bag in the refrigerator between pumping sessions. Pump pieces may need to be rinsed with water before storing if milk dries on the filters, but refrigeration may prevent the milk from drying. Consider what research has proven: breastmilk is safe at room temperature for several hours and in the refrigerator for 5-8 days (La Leche League International, 2008; Biagioli, 2003). Bacterial growth is retarded by both refrigeration and the nature of your milk.

The pieces of your pump that touch your milk (flanges, filters, bottles) will need to be washed with warm, soapy water at least once daily, preferably when you are at home. Some mothers also sterilize pump parts. This can be accomplished by boiling pump pieces briefly (check the manufacturer's instructions). A faster option is to purchase microwave-sterilizing bags. Most can be used multiple times. These bags can also be used to sterilize bottle nipples and pacifiers. The sterilization is effective in killing thrush strains.

Chapter 15
Your Baby's Day

Communication with your baby's childcare provider is important. You will need to take time to discuss routines, how your baby communicates, napping habits, and, of course, feeding. For some, communication will be strictly verbal. For others, written communication combined with verbal is preferred. Appendix E includes a sample feeding handout for you to fill in and share with your baby's caregiver, and a second feedback form for your caregiver to return to you. Receiving feedback will help you determine the correct quantity of milk and bottle nipple size as your baby grows.

Bottle Brand

Find out if your childcare provider uses the bottles provided by parents or if they construct generic bottles for feedings. You may need to specify that they use the bottles and bottle nipples you have carefully chosen.

First-Morning Bottle

If you are able to squeeze one pumping session in before leaving in the morning, ask your childcare provider to use the bottle of fresh, not refrigerated, breastmilk first (if stored at less than 77°).

Estimating Quantity

The amount of calories a baby needs is, in part, determined by the baby's weight and age. As a baby grows, the needed caloric intake gradually declines, which explains why the amount of milk a baby eats does not continuously increase throughout the first year. To get you started in knowing how much milk to leave for your baby, we have included an equation based on your baby's weight and eating schedule. It should be noted that this equation is based on formula intake; however, it provides a starting point.

You can estimate how much milk your baby is likely to take at each feeding by multiplying your baby's weight by 2.7, and then dividing that number by how many times your baby eats in a 24-hour day. This is how many ounces your baby is likely to eat at each feeding for the first few months. A chart of estimated quantity is included in Appendix F.

You need to be aware that solely breastfed infants often consume fewer calories and a lower volume of milk than formula-fed infants. Dr. Sears explains, "This doesn't mean that their mothers aren't producing enough milk. Instead, it's an indication that breastfed infants have an amazing ability to self-regulate their calorie intake according to their individual needs" (Sears, 2006b).

Every baby is different. Pay attention to your baby's feeding cues. Although charts may be helpful, they should be used as a general guideline. Keeping your baby's wellness appointments with his healthcare provider will help you know your baby is on track.

Avoiding Leftovers

After spending time and energy to pump and store your milk, it is important to use it carefully, wasting as little as possible. When your baby takes a bottle, ideally you will offer the amount of milk your baby is likely to eat. If your baby is still hungry, it is safest to pour some additional milk into the bottle to complete the feeding.

It is not widely recommended that breastmilk left in the bottle be saved for a later feeding because there are few studies to determine its safety. When a baby drinks from the bottle, the contents are exposed to germs. However, fresh breastmilk has properties that kill bacteria, whereas formula promotes bacterial growth.

Dr. Jim Sears writes, "Any milk that is left over after a feeding can be saved for the next feeding (just a few hours), otherwise you should discard it. The reason is that bacteria from the baby's mouth might have entered the bottle during feeding. This can lead to contamination if it sits too long" (Sears, 2006c). This is different than recommendations for formula use, which require that any amount left in the bottle needs to be discarded, since formula does not contain antibodies. This is a conversation you can have with your healthcare provider.

The breastfed baby is in control of how much he eats. Sometimes your baby may eat a little less than you thought, and sometimes your baby may want more. When a baby breastfeeds, we do not *make* a baby *finish* a feeding. When a breastfed baby drinks from a bottle, it is not necessary to *make* the baby *finish the bottle*. Some babies will eat part of a feeding, like an appetizer, and then want the "full course" a little while later. This is normal. However, if your baby is eating less than he has previously eaten on a consistent basis, perhaps it is time to move up in nipple size to a medium-flow nipple.

Less Than a Full Supply

Sometimes a mother will be unable to pump enough milk for a full feeding. Several remedies are possible. Your baby's caregiver can combine previously stored milk with the fresh milk to equal the amount your baby eats. This allows your baby to have the full benefits of fresh milk. If there is not any stored milk available to add, you can allow your baby's caregiver to add formula to the milk you have pumped to equal the amount your baby will eat. To be sure no breastmilk goes to waste, some mothers prefer the caregiver to give the baby the breastmilk first, and then offer a second bottle of formula.

When Milk Spills

Be mentally prepared—milk spills. This might happen when you are cleaning up from a pumping session. You might leave your pumped milk in the cooler pack over the weekend. Your husband or childcare giver might discard your breastmilk absent-mindedly. Take a deep breath. Yes, all your hard work and that portion of your baby's food are lost. It is sad, but it is not the end of the world.

If your milk is thrown out against your wishes, this needs to be addressed. Resist the urge to yell. Take a few moments to compose your thoughts. Explain what to do—storing and using—and then what not to do. Stating your point without accusations will help the listener to not feel defensive. The listener will be more likely to hear your concerns if you refrain from yelling, and perhaps this will pave the way to discuss solutions.

In the end, the relationships you have with your baby, husband, and childcare giver are more important than a few ounces of breastmilk. Keep your perspective, and let the knowledge that milk will spill inspire you to build a supply in the freezer during the early days.

Last Bottle at Daycare

It is important that you are able to feed your baby when you pick him up from daycare. Best-case scenario, feed your baby when you arrive to pick him up, before driving home. If your baby is hungry within an hour before your return and the caregiver offers a bottle of your milk, your baby will not be hungry when you pick him up, and your breasts will not be emptied. Not only will this make your breasts uncomfortable, but it puts your milk supply in jeopardy as well.

To avoid this common scenario, plan to send an "end-of-the-day" bottle with your baby, or keep a couple end-of-the-day bottles in their freezer.

This bottle will have 1-1½ ounces of breastmilk, just enough to keep your baby happy, but not enough to fill your baby up.

Some mothers separate their expressed milk to manipulate how full their babies feel throughout the day. The hindmilk (top layer), full of fat, is added to daytime bottles to help space feedings by offering extra fat to keep the baby feeling full (thus less bottle-feeding). The foremilk (lower layer) is saved for the end-of-the-day feeding, so the baby's thirst is quenched, but the baby will still be hungry. We do not recommend tinkering with the natural balance of foremilk and hindmilk your baby receives at each feeding without careful consideration and the assistance of a breastfeeding helper.

Instead of a partial bottle at the end of the day, another idea is to have your baby's caregiver offer the pacifier, if your baby uses one, before you arrive to help your baby wait to breastfeed. This is the only acceptable time a pacifier can be used to space feedings. Be respectful of your baby's cues. If the pacifier is not calming, an end-of-the-day bottle should be offered.

SECTION 5
Overcoming Obstacles

Chapter 16
Refusing the Breast or Bottle

After your baby learns to breastfeed and bottle-feed, he may be one of the many babies who willingly switches between breastfeeding and bottle-feeding and never complains. However, even when the bottle nipple or feeding system is chosen and introduced carefully, a baby might eventually fuss and prefer one method of feeding to the other. With patience and persistence, a refusing baby can be lovingly coaxed to accept the breast or bottle again.

Refusing the Breast

A nursing strike occurs when a breastfeeding baby suddenly refuses to breastfeed. Your comprehensive breastfeeding book will have a section on how to avoid and overcome a nursing strike. Unfortunately, the most prevalent suggestion is to avoid introducing and using a bottle nipple.

This has been stated in the literature because many times mothers have unknowingly picked bottle nipples that promoted a mouth placement, suck, or milk flow very different from breastfeeding. On occasion, a baby will have one normal sucking pattern. When this baby must learn two different techniques for sucking, he will choose the easiest, either breast or bottle, rejecting the other. This is called nipple preference. It can be very difficult to return to breastfeeding once nipple preference has occurred as a result of bottle-feeding with a nipple that creates poor mouth placement or flows too fast.

Rest assured that you can reduce the risk of this scenario by waiting to introduce a bottle until breastfeeding is well established (3-4 weeks old) and by choosing the bottle nipple according to the SIMPLE Method. Avoiding the bottle altogether is usually not an option if you are employed outside the home.

When a mother returns to work and her baby shifts from mostly breastfeeding to multiple bottle-feedings, the likelihood of a nursing strike may increase. If your baby is refusing the breast, first rule out sickness. Is he getting a cold? Is he teething or might he have thrush? Talk with your healthcare provider about medicinal comfort measures if you suspect illness. Next, consider your milk supply. Do you hear steady swallowing when your baby breastfeeds? Are you able to pump a full supply for his feedings? If you feel your supply is steady, you can devote your time to encouraging the breast. If you feel your milk supply is compromised, re-read the section "Boosting Your Milk Supply" in Chapter 13, so you can work on your supply while encouraging breastfeeding. Until your baby accepts the breast for all feedings when you are together, it will be important to use your pump for any missed feedings and supplement accordingly.

One approach to encourage breastfeeding is to increase skin-to-skin contact, meaning naked baby held against mother's naked chest. Taking a bath together works well for many mothers and babies. Remaining calm and talking sweetly to the baby are essential. Forcing a baby to breastfeed by jamming the breast in the baby's mouth is never kind and may actually prolong the nursing strike.

Refusing the Bottle

Two reasons a baby will refuse a bottle are late introduction and a bottle strike. Late introduction means the bottle is offered when the baby is past 3-4 weeks of age, as discussed in Chapter 9. By this time, the baby may have a strong preference for his mother's nipple and reject a bottle, called bottle nipple resistance.

A bottle strike occurs when a baby who formerly would take a bottle suddenly refuses. Very little has been written on this subject. Babies are unpredictable. Even with bottle practice, your baby may experience a bottle strike at some point. The good news is if you are reading this book from front to back, please feel confident that the occurrence of a bottle strike is greatly reduced.

A bottle strike often occurs with this sequence of events: a breastfeeding baby is introduced to a bottle nipple; the baby learns to accept the bottle; since the parents have discovered the best bottle nipple fit for their baby, they set it aside and resume total breastfeeds; the baby refuses the bottle when mother's maternity leave is over.

One distressed mother shared her dilemma: "I have a 3-month-old daughter who I have been solely breastfeeding. I will be returning to work full time in about 6 weeks, and my daughter refuses to take the bottle. She took the bottle in the first few weeks with no problem, but then we stopped, and now she will not take it. She cries frantically when the bottle is put to her lips and will continue to cry for as long as we try to feed her with it. I am really desperate and worried about returning to work."

Another panicked mother shared, "We first gave her the bottle at 6 or 7 weeks. She took it fine once or twice, but sometimes it was a struggle to get her to take it. We didn't really give her a bottle very often because I just tried to be here to feed her. I'm starting to get worried about taking her to the sitter! In hindsight, maybe we should have given her one more consistently." Bingo! Finding the best bottle nipple, then *practicing frequently*, is the best way to avoid a bottle strike. Breastfed babies prefer to *breastfeed*. Therefore, if you want to feel sure that your baby will bottle-feed when you are separated, practicing will bring security for you and familiarity for your baby. If you will be employed outside the home, we encourage daily practice. Reread page 79, which discusses practice schedules for various situations.

If you have waited past the 3-4-week recommended age of bottle introduction, there is still hope. Gentle, quiet encouragement and persistence will usually help older babies learn to accept a bottle. Facing the baby away from you with his back leaning against your chest may distract the unwilling baby (**Figure 16.1**). If your baby will not accept a bottle from you, another caregiver can offer the bottle while you are present to assess your baby's suck. If your baby will not accept the bottle while you are nearby, teach the caregiver the SIMPLE Method, so your baby's suck is as close to breastfeeding as possible.

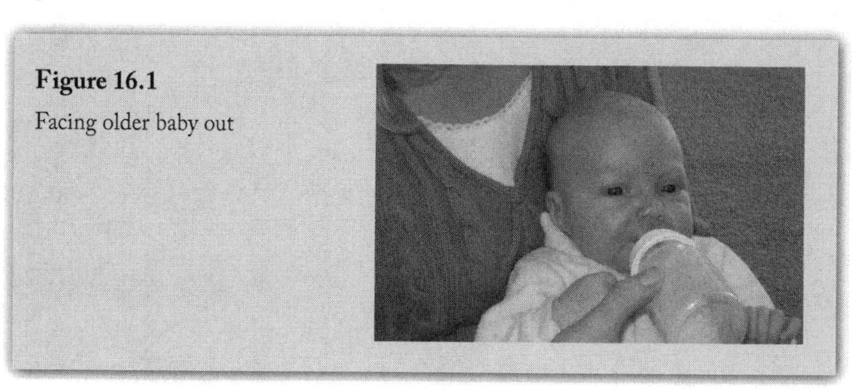

Figure 16.1

Facing older baby out

Even if you have diligently helped your baby practice feeding with the bottle, a bottle strike can occur at any time. A common age for a strike is when your baby is three months old, when developmentally babies become more aware.

Similar principles to overcoming a nursing strike can be applied to overcoming a bottle-strike. The most important point is the parents' attitude—if the baby perceives taking the bottle with frustration and panic from a parent, the baby will mirror frustration and panic. Before trying the techniques, there are some basic rules that apply before your problem solving begins.

The rules:

- Rule out physical problems: earache, cold, thrush, teething.
- Breathe. Relax. Smile. Breathe some more.
- Make bottle-time playtime. Letting your baby happily mouth the nipple is a good step in future acceptance.
- Offer the bottle at least twice a day during the "strike," preferably when everyone is happy and relaxed. For most families, this is morning time when the baby is happy and when the mother has the highest level of "mother" hormones.
- Practice for 10-15 minutes with your baby, doing your best to keep everyone happy.
- If your baby becomes sad, do not breastfeed right away. Instead, comfort and distract your baby, then breastfeed about 10 minutes later, so your baby does not associate refusing the bottle with winning the breast.
- When your baby *does* accept the bottle and will eat about 2 ounces, it is okay to finish the feeding with breastfeeding.
- If you have already found the best bottle nipple "fit" as suggested in Chapter 6, it is not necessary to purchase more bottle nipple varieties. Consistency in offering the nipple you have is a better choice.

Many techniques to encourage taking the bottle use distraction, a few involve trickery. What works with one baby may not work with another, so we have gathered a host of ideas to encourage your baby to accept the bottle. You can change a baby's environment and input in many ways to encourage a successful bottle-feeding. Give each idea you try two or three feedings to work before trying another idea.

Position

- If your baby will accept the bottle from mom, but not from dad, try handing the baby off during a feeding and offering the bottle "together."
- Try different feeding positions in your arms: baby's back leaning on adult's chest, baby "sitting" on adult's lap, baby facing adult.
- Try different feeding positions while *not* being held: in the baby swing, in a bouncy chair, on the couch, in a stroller, in the car seat.

Location

- Feed outside while looking at the trees, bushes, or clouds (try both in your arms and out of your arms).
- Choose a place to bottle-feed where your baby does not breastfeed (not the rocker or nursing "corner").
- Introduce the bottle while your baby is in the bath.

Timing

- Offer the bottle about 30 minutes after breastfeeding, when your baby is awake, but not hungry.
- Offer the bottle when your baby shows signs of being hungry.
- Offer the bottle when your baby awakens from a nap, still slightly groggy and wanting to breastfeed.
- Offer the bottle for a middle-of-the-night feeding using one of the following strategies: start with a bottle at the beginning of a feeding, switching to breastfeeding after baby eats an ounce; or start with breastfeeding and after the first let-down at the breast, finish the feeding with the bottle.

Associations & Distractions

- Sing the same song at each feeding time: sing to your baby before you feed, and sing once more while you feed. Singing while you breastfeed may help your baby associate this song with feeding from the bottle. This association can transfer between mom, dad, and caregiver.
- Hide the bottle with a small blanket, washcloth (**Figure 16.2**), or stuffed animal. When you find a cover you and your baby prefer, continue to use the same bottle "cover" for association. Consider buying a stack of washcloths (the same color) to send with your baby to daycare for consistency, and to double as a burp cloth (hence, more than one).
- Swaddle your baby in a blanket or piece of clothing (nightshirt) that smells like mom.

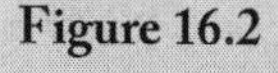

Figure 16.2

Distracting baby in bath with a wash cloth hiding the bottle

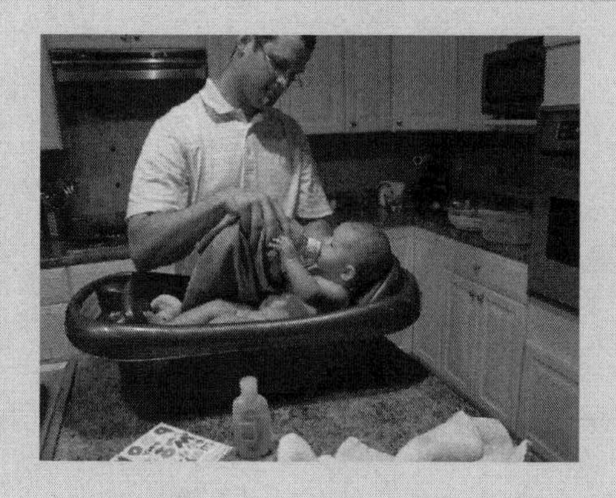

Nipple Switch

- While your baby nurses to sleep, remove your nipple from the baby's mouth and replace it with the bottle nipple.
- While your baby is nursing during a wakeful time of day, try replacing your nipple with the bottle *after* the first let-down, so your baby's initial hunger is satisfied with breastfeeding.
- If your baby uses a pacifier, try replacing the pacifier with the bottle nipple.
- If your baby is willing to suck on your finger, slip the bottle in while the baby is sucking. This will affect the mouth placement temporarily, but might get the baby over the hump.

Other Points to Consider

- If your baby is older than 3-4 months, be sure he is willing to accept things other than the breast in his mouth: teether toys, blankies, stuffed animals, washcloths, etc.

Do Not

- *Do not* engage in bottle battles that involve a screaming baby and a frustrated daddy—your baby needs to associate his dad with happy activities. If interaction with dad is saved for learning to bottle-feed, your baby might think his daddy is the cause of sadness.
- *Do not* let the baby get "good and hungry," so he takes the bottle—this is a very harsh idea. There are numerous *kind* ways to encourage your baby to take a bottle, rather than starving him.
- *Do not* replace breastmilk with formula or juice thinking perhaps the baby does not want to taste breastmilk from a different source. This is not a good idea because this jeopardizes the lining of your baby's intestines, sets your baby up for tummy woes, and exposes your baby to early allergens.
- *Do not* let the caregiver figure out how to feed your baby—leaving your baby can feel worrisome in itself; adding the layer of, "Will my baby eat?" creates more stress.
- *Do not* plan to feed your baby long-term with a syringe, eye-dropper, or medicine cup—babies like and need to suck. If you will be away from your baby for several feedings in a row, finding a bottle your baby will take can make everyone happier: baby, caregiver, and parents.
- *Do not* switch to a higher flow nipple—pouring milk into your baby's mouth is essentially force feeding, creating an unhappy experience and a risk for aspiration and choking.

Share this checklist with your baby's caregiver if your baby is reluctant to take a bottle when you are apart. A copy is included in Appendix G.

A breast or bottle strike comes unexpectedly, with a mother's panic following. Knowing there are many ways to lovingly encourage your baby to eat can help remove this stress. You can breathe a sigh of relief when your baby accepts the breast, or bottle, again.

Chapter 17
Sleep Like a Baby

Sleep like a baby is an oxymoron! Most healthy newborns awaken every 2 to 3 hours, 24 hours a day, to eat. For some babies, this pattern of waking during the night continues for many months.

Quite often, a baby will have at least one longer sleep stretch. It can be tempting to let your baby have a longer sleep period during the day, so you can get things done. Try and resist this temptation, and save the longer sleep stretch for the night. Instead, awaken your baby for frequent daytime feedings, and perhaps he will sleep longer at night.

It is uncommon for young babies to sleep for eight hours at night. "Easy" babies who sleep this long usually become "normal" babies around four months of age, and begin waking at frequent intervals to eat. This is to be expected.

The medical definition of "sleeping through the night" is five hours. A baby who goes to sleep at 9:00 PM and awakens at 2:00 AM has slept through the night. After this longer stretch, a baby will then begin to awaken at more frequent intervals to eat. While this may seem tiring and overwhelming to read, it is important to have a realistic viewpoint of "normal."

Some families find it is easy to breastfeed at night because there are no bottles to prepare or breastmilk to pump. Sleeping in close proximity to the baby can simplify feedings. Responding to the baby's feeding cues promptly will help the baby stay drowsy and return to sleep easier. Also, sometimes a mother breastfeeds her baby lying down in bed, so she feels rested.

Night feedings are important. If you are hoping to have a long stretch of sleep, it is important that your baby feeds a lot during the day. For example, those three night feedings you wish to avoid need to be moved to three *additional* feedings during the day, preferably one at a time; they cannot simply be omitted. However, a baby should not be forced to eat more than he is willing to eat, so this may or may not work.

Sometimes a baby will want to sleep at the childcare center, without eating, and breastfeed frequently throughout the night when he is with his mother. This is normal for some babies. Pryor (1997) calls this reverse-cycle feeding. Some mothers who work find that bringing the baby to bed at night helps them feel close to the baby and lets the baby eat a lot while they are together. This is an acceptable choice and works well for some families.

In some situations, sleep becomes a needed priority. Mothers who work outside the home or mothers whose health and wellness is dependent upon rest may choose to limit their involvement during the night. Often the father takes over nighttime caretaking and feedings. Ideally, breastmilk is in the bottle, and you will need to pump for that feeding. If you have a plentiful milk supply, consider pumping before bed (after your baby's last feeding) and save that milk for the nighttime feeding. Some moms use the breastmilk pumped earlier in the day or borrow from the freezer supply. If you fall short for a full feeding, add another type of baby milk to the breastmilk to equal the feeding (Chapter 12). Do not let the baby sleep with the bottle because of potential tooth decay and risk of choking. Take the bottle away before you lay your baby down.

The subject of "how" to put a baby to sleep is also significant. The scientific mechanism is not fully understood, but sucking is associated with a reduced risk of SIDS. The American Academy of Pediatrics (AAP) Task Force on Sudden Infant Death Syndrome (2005, p. 1252) suggests to "consider offering a pacifier at nap time and bedtime" throughout the first year of life, after breastfeeding is established (3-4 weeks old). From birth through the first birthday, there is a protective measure against SIDS when a baby sucks as he drifts off to sleep. It is okay to breastfeed your baby to sleep. Babies who are breastfeeding as they go to sleep are already sucking. When a baby goes to sleep *without* breastfeeding, such as when a baby is at daycare or when a mother works the night shift, a pacifier can add that element of protection.

The AAP Task Force also recommends, "The pacifier should be used when placing the infant down for sleep and not be reinserted once the infant falls asleep. If the infant refuses the pacifier, he or she should not be forced to take it" (2005, p. 1252). They do not suggest removing the baby from the breast at the end of a feeding to take a pacifier. They do not suggest putting a pacifier into the mouth of a baby who is sleeping. They do not suggest that babies who do not want a pacifier need one.

If you use a pacifier to help your baby go to sleep, we still encourage weaning from daytime pacifier use when your baby is 4 months old, and total pacifier weaning at one year.

Clearly, there are many considerations in meeting your baby's nighttime needs. Most babies eat at least once during the night. Thankfully, balancing sleep and night feedings is temporary because your baby will soon outgrow this stage. Books entirely devoted to this topic are available. Some of our favorites are *Good Nights* by Dr. Jay Gordon, *The No Cry Sleep Solution Book* by Elizabeth Pantley, and *Nighttime Parenting* by Dr. William Sears.

Chapter 18
Ways to Delay Weaning

Weaning can be many things. Usually, it means to discontinue use of breast, bottle, or pacifier. In Chapter 1, you learned that weaning from the breast is a personal decision guided by the recommendations of healthcare organizations. In Chapters 9 and 10, you learned guidelines for when to wean from the bottle and pacifier.

Let's recap what you have read thus far, looking at weaning times from earliest to latest.

- Pacifier daytime use: 4 months old
- Pacifier nap or nighttime use: 12 months old
- Bottle: 12-18 months old
- Breast: at least a year, and longer as mutually desired (AAP, 2005) two years or longer (WHO, 2009)

Since babies are meant to breastfeed for at least a year, why do so many babies wean before their birthday? There are certain developmental stages that are sometimes misinterpreted as weaning. Also, many mothers are ready to wean before their baby's first birthday. Let's explore both.

The primary reason for premature weaning is misinterpreting a growth spurt. As discussed in Chapter 2, babies have growth spurts when they nurse frequently for several days, which boosts moms' milk supply. Many mothers think they do not have enough milk when the baby nurses "nonstop" for 2 or 3 days, and elect to wean. Non-stop nursing for 2 or 3 days is a normal phenomenon. With unlimited access to the breast for this short time period, the milk supply increases and the feeding intervals space again. If you are employed outside the home, this means you will need to nurse more frequently when you and your baby are together to boost your supply. You might also want to consider adding an additional pumping session during a growth spurt.

If your milk supply is truly low, you can continue breastfeeding while building your milk supply, rather than weaning. Refer to Chapter 13 for ideas on ways to increase your supply. Help from your healthcare provider and/or a breastfeeding helper (Appendix B) may be necessary.

Around 4 to 6 months of age, many babies become social. Along with this awareness of what is going on around them comes distraction. This does not mean the baby is no longer interested in nursing and ready to wean. A baby of this age likes to pull off the breast and see what he is missing, often leaving milk spraying everywhere but in his mouth. This is a normal stage. Sometimes these babies make up for the feedings they miss by breastfeeding more frequently at night. If your baby prefers to look around instead of eat, you might need to feed your baby in a quiet, dark, boring room.

Biting is not an indication that your baby is ready to wean. When a baby is breastfeeding correctly, his tongue covers his lower teeth (or gum ridge) and inhibits the biting reflex. However, many mothers experience biting at some point while they are breastfeeding. Babies bite for different reasons. If your baby bites, you will probably notice a pattern of when it happens. When a baby falls asleep nursing, the tongue may slip back off the lower gum ridge, triggering the baby to clamp down. Keeping your finger "at the ready" to unlatch a sleeping baby will prevent biting in this circumstance. Some babies who are teething bite at the beginning of a feeding or perhaps when the milk flow slows. Offering the baby an acceptable teething object before a feeding or anticipating the switch from nutritive to non-nutritive sucking will discourage biting. If you struggle with a biting baby, contact a breastfeeding helper for further suggestions before considering weaning.

Occasionally a baby will cry at the breast and not want to feed. Babies do not cry because they want to wean. Instead, teething, ear infections, sore throat, or thrush can make a baby feel uncomfortable because his mouth hurts. It is important to figure out what is causing the unhappiness and work through the problem. Calling a breastfeeding helper (Appendix B) is often the fastest way to resume breastfeeding.

Many mothers wish to wean for nighttime feedings before the baby's first birthday, but continue daytime feedings. Unfortunately, breastfeeding at night and during sleep are usually the last to go. As mentioned in Chapter 17, *Sleep Like a Baby*, if you wish to reduce nighttime feedings, make sure your baby is feeding more often during the day. To learn more about nighttime weaning, some helpful books are *Good Nights* by Dr. Jay Gordon and *The No Cry Sleep Solution Book* by Elizabeth Pantley.

Life's circumstances can influence the decision to wean. Let's consider how to balance breastfeeding, separation, milk supply, and weaning. There are many scenarios.

Being unable to pump enough milk for feedings does not warrant weaning. It is safe to mix the milk you pumped with breastmilk you saved earlier in the same bottle. If you do not have any extra breastmilk saved, you can use the milk you have pumped and add another appropriate baby milk to equal the amount your baby normally eats. Refer to the *Strategy's* list of baby milk choices in Chapter 1. *Some* breastmilk is healthier than *no* breastmilk.

Some mothers are unable to pump at work and wonder if they should wean altogether, since the baby will be eating formula during the day. It is healthier to continue breastfeeding when you are with your baby. *Some* breastmilk is healthier than *no* breastmilk.

Sometimes a mother may feel overwhelmed, too busy to cope with the many tasks of mothering, working, and running a household, and decide to wean her baby. Before making this decision, understand that breastfeeding does not need to be an all-or-nothing venture. Will replacing one feeding give you enough time to gain some control? Have you considered breastfeeding during daylight hours and bottle-feeding at night? Or the opposite? Your baby must eat, and you will continue to hold and love your baby, regardless of your feeding method. You and your baby will benefit when you are able to maintain some breastfeeding. Try to find a balance that allows for partial breastfeeding.

The definition of weaning means to be fulfilled or to gradually remove some favored object. Mothers and babies wean at different times, for different reasons. The preferred time is after the first birthday. The preferred way is to wean slowly over a few weeks, rather than a one-time event. Whatever time works for your family, we hope you and your baby come to a place of mutual fulfillment.

Epilogue
Of Monkeys and Mothers

In 1958, a scientist named Harry Harlow conducted a study using monkeys he called, "The Nature of Love." Harlow studied the importance of contact comfort and nursing comfort of baby monkeys using two surrogate mother monkeys. One was a bare welded wire cylindrical form surmounted by a wooden head with a crude face. The other welded wire form was cushioned with sponge rubber and a sheathing of terry cloth. Both "mothers" had a light bulb behind them radiating heat. Harlow placed eight newborn monkeys in individual cages, each with equal access to a cloth and a wire mother. Four of the infants received their milk from the wire monkey, and four from the cloth monkey. Regardless of which mother monkey the baby monkeys received their milk from, both groups of monkeys chose to spend their non-eating time on the soft cloth mothers.

Harlow also exposed the baby monkeys to emotional stress in the form of a mechanical teddy bear which moved forward, beating a drum. Whether the infants had nursed from the wire or the cloth mother, they always sought comfort from their soft cloth mother. Harlow summarized his findings by discussing the importance of contact comfort in the development of infant affection. This study highlights how the emotional attachment of the baby monkeys rested largely upon access to a nearby, soft "mother," regardless of how the baby monkeys received their milk.

We end our book with this study to highlight the importance of emotional attachment. Like baby monkeys, the emotional attachment of human babies is dependent on nurturing and physical attachment. Attachment is more than just providing your baby with breastmilk. Your baby will flourish when you are available to him on all levels—mentally, emotionally, and physically.

The many demands of motherhood can feel daunting and draining regardless of where you work, whether inside or outside the home. With mothers typically shouldering the brunt of running a household and ensuring their babies are getting enough milk, it is no wonder many mothers become overwhelmed. If you feel overwhelmed or become consumed with breastfeeding or pumping, and no longer want to hold, love, and enjoy your baby, something needs to change. Changing one or two small things can help you avoid feeling resentful towards your baby. Here are some ideas mothers have shared with us:

- The housework really can wait—it will be there tomorrow, next week, and even next year.
- If meal preparation is discouraging, use a crock-pot and double recipes so you can have leftovers.
- Rely more on friends and family for carpooling and errands.
- Reduce extra-curricular activities and volunteer time.
- Rethink your priorities.

Breastfeeding need not be all-or-none. Breastfeeding can range from exclusive, to nursing just for comfort, with many combinations in between. Even replacing just one breastfeeding with a bottle can make all the difference and help you enjoy your baby and reach your breastfeeding goals. Choose what is best for you, your family, and your situation. Remember, your baby needs a soft mother, not a wire monkey.

References

Alekseev, N.P., Ilyin, V.I., Yaroslavski, V.K., Gaidukov, S.N., Tikhonova, T.K., Specivcev, Y.A., et al. (1998). Compression stimuli increase the efficacy of breast pump function. *European Journal of Obstetrics Gynecology and Reproductive Biology, 77*(2), 131-139.

American Academy of Pediatrics. (1998). *Caring for your baby and young child birth to age 5.* New York: Bantam Books.

American Academy of Pediatrics Section on Breastfeeding. (2005). Breastfeeding and the use of human milk. *Pediatrics, 115*(2), 496-506.

American Academy of Pediatrics, Task Force on Sudden Infant Death Syndrome. (2005). The changing concept of sudden infant death syndrome: diagnostic coding shifts, controversies regarding the sleeping environment, and new variables to consider in reducing risk. *Pediatrics, 116*(5), 1245-1255.

Beckman, D. (2000, November). Oral motor assessment and intervention [Conference]. Salt Lake City, Utah.

Biagioli, F. (2003). Returning to work while breastfeeding. *American Family Physician, 68*(11), 2201-2208.

Bonyata, K. (2007). Method used by Kellymom.com to calculate average weight gain per week using the WHO Child Growth Standards. Retrieved January 15, 2009, from http://www.kellymom.com/babyconcerns/growth/avg-wt-gain-calculations.pdf.

Colburn-Smith, C., & Serette, A. (2007). *The milk memos: How real moms learned to mix business with babies—and how you can, too.* New York: Penguin Group.

Colson, S.D., Meek, J.H., & Hawdon, J.M. (2008). Optimal positions for the release of primitive neonatal reflexes stimulating breastfeeding. *Early Human Development, 84*, 441-449.

Cotterman, K.J. (2004). Reverse pressure softening: a simple tool to prepare areola for easier latching during engorgement. *Journal of Human Lactation, 20*, 227-237.

Ezz El Din, Z.M., Abd El Ghaffar, S., El Gabry, E.K., Fahmi, W.A., & Bedair, R.F. (2004). Is stored expressed breastmilk an alternative for working Egyptian mothers? *East Mediterranean Health Journal, 10*(6), 815-821.

Food and Drug Administration (FDA). (2009). Should I buy a used breast pump or share a breast pump? Retrieved September 18, 2009 from http://www.fda.gov/MedicalDevices/ProductsandMedicalProcedures/HomeHealthandConsumer/ConsumerProducts/BreastPumps/ucm061939.htm.

Geddes, D.T. (2009). The use of ultrasound to identify milk ejection in women—tips and pitfalls. *International Breastfeeding Journal, 4*(5), published online June 1, 2009, http://www.internationalbreastfeedingjournal.com/content/4/1/5.

Hanna, N., Ahmed, K., Anwar, M., Petrova, A., Hiatt, M., & Hegyi, T. (2004). Effect of storage on breastmilk antioxidant activity. *Archives of Disease in Childhood, Fetal and Neonatal Edition, 89*(6), F518-F520.

Harlow, H.F. (1959). Love in infant monkeys. *Scientific American, 200*(6), 64-74.

Howard, C.R., Howard, F.M., Lanphear, B., Eberly, S., deBlieck, E.A., Oakes, D., & Lawrence, R.A. (2003). Randomized clinical trial of pacifier use and bottle-feeding or cupfeeding and their effect on breastfeeding. *Pediatrics, 111*(3), 511-518.

Ip, S., Chung, M., Raman, G., Chew, P., Magula, N., DeVine, D., et al. (2007). Breastfeeding and maternal and infant health outcomes in developed countries, structured abstract. *Agency for Healthcare Research and Quality.* Retrieved August 1, 2008, from http://www.ahrq.gov/clinic/tp/brfouttp.htm.

Karp, H. (2003). *The happiest baby on the block.* New York: Bantam Books.

Kent, J.C., Ramsay, D.T., Doherty, D., Larsson, M., & Hartmann, P.E. (2003). Response of breasts to different stimulation patterns of an electric breast pump. *Journal of Human Lactation, 19*(2), 179-186.

La Leche League International. (2008). *Storing human milk* (No. 10134). Schaumburg, Illinois: Author.

La Leche League International. (2004). *The womanly art of breastfeeding.* Schaumburg, Illinois: Author.

Lawrence, R.A., & Lawrence, R.M. (1999). *Breastfeeding: a guide for the medical professional.* St. Louis: Mosby.

Matthew, O.P. (1988). Nipple units for newborn infants: a functional comparison. *Pediatrics, 81*(5), 688-691.

Mattos-Graner, R.O., de Moraes, A.B., Rontani, R.M., & Birman, E.G. (2001). Relation of oral yeast infection in Brazilian infants and use of a pacifier. *ASDC Journal of Dentistry for Children, 68*(1), 33-36, 10.

Mitoulas, L.R., Lai, C.T., Gurrin, L.C., Larsson, M., & Hartmann, P.E. (2002). Efficacy of breastmilk expression using an electric breast pump. *Journal of Human Lactation, 18*(4), 344-352.

Mizuno, K., & Ueda, A. (2006). Changes in sucking performance from nonnutritive sucking to nutritive sucking during breast- and bottle–feeding. *Pediatric Research, 59*(5), 728-731.

Mohrbacher, N., & Stock, J. (2003). *The breastfeeding answer book.* Schaumburg, Illinois: La Leche League International.

North, K., Fleming, P, Golding, J., & the Avon Longitudinal Study of Pregnancy and Childhood Study Team. (1999). Pacifier use and morbidity in the first six months of life. *Pediatrics, 103*(3), e34.

Nowak, A.J., Smith, W.L., & Erenberg, A. (1994). Imaging evaluation of artificial nipples during bottle-feeding. *Archives of Pediatrics & Adolescent Medicine, 148,* 40-42.

Nowak, A.J., Smith, W.L., & Erenberg, A. (1995). Imaging evaluation of breast-feeding and bottle-feeding systems. *Journal of Pediatrics, 126*(6), 130-134.

Pryor, G. (1997). *Nursing mother, working mother.* Boston: The Harvard Common Press.

Ransjo-Arvidson, A.B., Matthiesen, A.S., Lilja, G., Nissen, E., Widstrom, A.M., & Uvnas-Moberg, K. (2001). Maternal analgesia during labor disturbs newborn behavior: effects on breastfeeding, temperature, and crying. *Birth, 28,* 5-12.

Reder, A., Catalfo, P., & Renfrow Hamilton, S. (1999). *The whole parenting guide.* New York: Broadway Books.

Riordan, J., & Wambach, K. (2010). *Breastfeeding and human lactation,* 4th ed. Sudbury, Massachusetts: Jones and Bartlett Publishers.

Sears, J. (2006c). *Reusing breastmilk.* Retrieved August 5, 2008, from http://www.askdrsears.com/faq/bf28.asp.

Sears, W., & Sears, M. (1993). *The baby book.* Boston: Little, Brown and Company.

Sears, W. (2006a). *Ear infections.* Retrieved October, 8, 2008, from http://www.askdrsears.com/html/8/t081600.asp.

Sears, W. (2006b). *Weight gain growth patterns.* Retrieved October, 8, 2008, from http://www.askdrsears.com/html/2/t023600.asp.

Sexton, S., & Natale, R. (2009). Risks and benefits of pacifiers. *American Family Physician, 79*(8), 681-685.

Smillie, C.M. (2008). How infants learn to feed: a neurobehavioral model. In C.W. Genna (Ed.). *Supporting sucking skills in breastfeeding infants* (pp. 79-95). Sudbury, MA: Jones & Bartlett Publishers.

Smith, L.J. (1998). *Don't shake the milk.* Retrieved February 12, 2008, from http://www.bflrc.com/ljs/breastfeeding/shakenot.htm.

Soares, M.E., Giugliani, E.R., Braun, M.L., Salgado, A.C., de Oliveira, A.P., & de Aguiar, P.R. (2003). Pacifier use and its relationship with early weaning in infants born at a child-friendly hospital (translated). *Journal of Pediatrics (Rio J), 79*(4), 309-316.

Tully, M.R. (2000). Recommendations for handling of mother's own milk. *Journal of Human Lactation, 16,* 149-151.

United States Breastfeeding Committee. (2002). Economic benefits of breastfeeding (Issue paper). Raleigh, NC: Author.

Walker, M. (2001). *Selling out mothers and babies: marketing of breastmilk substitutes.* Weston, MA: National Alliance for Breastfeeding Advocacy.

West, D., & Marasco, L. (2009). *The breastfeeding mother's guide to making more milk.* New York: Mc-Graw-Hill.

Williamson, M.T., & Murti, P.K. (1996). Effects of storage, time, temperature, and composition of containers on biologic components of human milk. *Journal of Human Lactation, 12*(1), 31-35.

World Health Organization. (2003). *Global strategy for infant and young child feeding.* Singapore: Author.

World Health Organization. (2009). *Infant and young child feeding: model chapter for textbooks for medical students and allied health professionals.* France: Author.

World Health Organization Child Growth Standards. (2006). Retrieved January 15, 2009, from http://www.who.int/childgrowth/en/.

APPENDICES

Appendix A
Recommended Breastfeeding Books

Breastfeeding Made Simple: Seven Natural Laws for Nursing Mothers by Nancy Mohrbacher, IBCLC, and Kathleen Kendall-Tackett, PhD, IBCLC

The Ultimate Breastfeeding Book of Answers by Jack Newman, MD, and Teresa Pitman

The Womanly Art of Breastfeeding by La Leche League International

The Breastfeeding Mother's Guide to Making More Milk by Diana West, IBCLC, and Lisa Marasco, IBCLC

The Latch by Jack Newman, MD, and Teresa Pitman

25 Things Every New Mother Should Know by Martha Sears, RN, and William Sears, MD

Good Nights by Jay Gordon, MD

The No Cry Sleep Solution by Elizabeth Pantley

Nighttime Parenting by William Sears, MD

Appendix B
Breastfeeding Helpers

Different titles reflect various levels of training. Ask your helper what type of training she has received, how recently she received it, and how often she updates her knowledge. In many instances, correct titles are misused. New research is changing breastfeeding management. What was thought to be the best management strategy 10-15 years ago has been replaced with newer evidence-based support. Breastfeeding helpers need to frequently update their knowledge to keep on top of the latest information. If the first breastfeeding helper you meet with cannot answer your questions or if your problems do not improve in a day or so, contact another, more knowledgeable helper. The following are some terms used by breastfeeding helpers:

- **IBCLC**—International Board Certified Lactation Consultant—Also called a lactation consultant, this person is a breastfeeding professional with the highest level of knowledge and skill in breastfeeding support. If the person has IBCLC after their name, she/he has passed an international credentialing exam. To be eligible to take the exam, the individual must have extensive training and years of experience working with breastfeeding mothers. Many lactation consultants work in hospitals, birthing centers, and clinics. Many are in private practice. They usually charge for their services. Lactation consultants may also be a doctor, nurse, dietitian, speech therapist, etc. They may have various areas of expertise, so it might be advisable to work with more than one if you encounter difficult problems. Visit the website www.ILCA.org to find the IBCLC nearest you.
- **Lactation Educator/Counselor**—is an individual who has taken one or more breastfeeding courses. She/he can teach mothers about breastfeeding and help with normal problems. Some of these individuals may be certified by a local or national organization. These individuals may or may not have the expertise and experience to solve difficult problems. They may work in hospitals, birthing centers, and clinics. They may also be a nurse, dietitian, speech therapist, etc.
- **La Leche League Leader**—is a mother who started as a La Leche League member. After participating in extensive coursework and an accreditation process, she has become a La Leche League leader.

These mothers volunteer their time and effort to help other mothers successfully breastfeed. They provide peer support by facilitating monthly La Leche League classes, providing counseling, and providing telephone support. Visit the website www.LLLI.org to find a group or leader near you.

- **WIC Peer Counselor** –is a mother who is on (or has been on) the WIC program (Special Supplemental Food Program for Women, Infants, and Children) and has successfully breastfed her baby. She has gone through an extensive training program and provides peer support by teaching new moms about breastfeeding and helping with normal problems. Some WIC peer counselors work in WIC offices. Others visit new moms in the hospital. Some even make home visits.

Appendix C
"Slow-Flow" Rankings

Using a hospital grade breast pump, we tested and categorized various brands of slow flow nipples as very-slow, medium-slow, and fast-slow. We suggest "very-slow" is too slow for most babies, while "fast-slow" is too fast for most babies. Within each category, brands are listed from slowest to fastest flow. We recognize that vacuum is only one component of a baby's suck, and that flow may also vary with compression.

Very-slow:

Dr. Brown's Ultra Premie
Dr. Brown's Narrow Premie
OrganicKidz™ Narrow
Comotomo ™
Milk Bank™
Playtex® Petite VentAire®
Playtex® Petite Nurser Drop-Ins™
Playtex® Fullsized VentAire®
Playtex® Fullsized Nurser Drop-Ins™

Medium-slow:

Dr. Brown's Narrow Level 1
Dr. Brown's Wide
Munchkin® LATCH™
Similac Pink (hospital)
Evenflo® Proflow™ Narrow
Playtex® Angled VentAire®
Playtex® Angled Nurser Drop-Ins™
Playtex® Breastlike Shape VentAire®
Playtex® Breastlike Shape Nurser Drop-Ins™
Playtex® NaturaLatch® VentAire®
Playtex® NaturaLatch® Nurser Drop-Ins™
Enfamil Slow Flow (hospital)
Similac® SimplySmart™
Born Free™
Evenflo® Classic™ Silicone

Joovy® Boob
Avent Classic
Avent Natural Newborn flow 0m+
TruVent™ Evenflo
Lansinoh® mOmma
Medela® ("Wide")
MAM
Mimijumi
Nuby™ Parent's Choice
Tommee Tippee®
Gerber® Nuk Orthodontic Narrow, Silicone

Fast-slow:

Gerber® Nuk® Orthodontic Narrow, Latex
Similac brown (hospital)
Evenflo® Proflow™ Wide Bebek®
OrganicKidz™ Wide
Gerber® Nuk® Orthodontic Wide
Avent Natural Slow Flow 1m+
Medela Calma®

Excluded:

Two brands were excluded from the above list because their flow rates varied too greatly: Breastflow™ and MeadJohnson Hospital nuk

Two brands were excluded because the flow is dependent upon compression, which could not be controlled in our study: Nuby™ Non-Drip and Prince Lionheart®

Two brands were excluded because the nipple shape could not be tested with our equipment: Kiinde™ and Evenflo® Zoo Friends™ Anatomic Nipple

Appendix D
Checklist for Work

Items for Mom's pump bag:

- Breast pump with all parts and tubing
- Extra filters/membranes: one set attached to your breast pump, an extra set stored in your bag
- Two 4-ounce bottles or collection bags for <u>each</u> pumping session
- Power supply: extension cord, extra batteries
- Ice packs and tote, or refrigerator container
- Nursing pads if your breasts leak
- Cleaning method of choice
- Baby mementos: picture, blanket (optional)
- Hands-free bustier (optional)
- Nursing CD/MP3 (optional)

Appendix E
Communication with Child Care Provider

How to Feed My Baby

My Baby: ______________________ Age:________

1. Brand of nipple and/or feeding system my baby uses:__________________

2. Counting from the beginning of a feeding, my baby usually eats every ______ hours. When s/he roots and eats his hands, feel free to feed him if s/he is hungry.

3. Gently swirl the bottle of milk before feeding the baby to redistribute fat in the milk. Do not shake the breastmilk.

4. If I have time to pump before bringing my baby, you will find my baby's first bottle stored in the diaper bag at room temperature. Please do not refrigerate this first bottle.

5. Other bottles need to be refrigerated or frozen until feeding time.

6. To defrost a bottle of milk, please
   - ❑ hold the bottle under warm (not hot) water
   - ❑ place in a dish of warm water 30 minutes before a feeding
   - ❑ use the bottle warmer I provided

7. It is / is not necessary to warm my baby's bottle.

8. My baby eats about ________ ounces for daytime feedings. If my baby would like more, please pour 1 additional ounce of breastmilk into the bottle to offer.

9. If my baby does not finish a feeding, please:
   - ❑ discard
   - ❑ put the bottle in the refrigerator and offer it again within four hours; discard if the next feeding is after four hours.

10. If my baby would like a bottle within one hour of being picked up, please offer a smaller quantity "end-of-the-day" bottle.

My Baby Ate Journal

Please fill in this journal on the days circled because it will help me send the right amount of milk, and also let me know when it is time to adjust my baby's nipple size.

Baby's name:______________________

Monday	Time offered	How long feeding lasted	Amount eaten	Leftovers	Amount added
1st feeding					
2nd feeding					
3rd feeding					
4th feeding					

Comments:

Tuesday	Time offered	How long feeding lasted	Amount eaten	Leftovers	Amount added
1st feeding					
2nd feeding					
3rd feeding					
4th feeding					

Comments:

Wednesday	Time offered	How long feeding lasted	Amount eaten	Leftovers	Amount added
1st feeding					
2nd feeding					
3rd feeding					
4th feeding					

Comments:

Thursday	Time offered	How long feeding lasted	Amount eaten	Leftovers	Amount added
1st feeding					
2nd feeding					
3rd feeding					
4th feeding					

Comments:

Friday	Time offered	How long feeding lasted	Amount eaten	Leftovers	Amount added
1st feeding					
2nd feeding					
3rd feeding					
4th feeding					

Comments:

Appendix F
Estimated Quantity of Breastmilk

The weights listed increase by ½ pound increments. Find the weight closest to your baby's weight (column 1). Divide the total number of ounces (column 2) by the number of times your baby usually eats in 24 hours. The answer is approximately how much milk your baby is likely to eat from a bottle (insert into column 3).

Pounds	Total ounces of breastmilk in 24 hours	Divide total ounces by your baby's number of feedings to determine estimated quantity
8	21.6	
8.5	23	
9	24.3	
9.5	25.7	
10	27	
10.5	28.4	
11	29.7	
11.5	31	
12	32.4	
12.5	33.8	
13	35.1	

Appendix G
Checklist for Overcoming a Bottle Nipple Strike

The rules:

- Rule out physical problems: earache, cold, thrush, teething.
- Breathe. Relax. Smile. Breathe some more.
- Make bottle-time playtime. Letting your baby happily mouth the nipple is a good step in future acceptance.
- Offer the bottle at least twice a day during the "strike," preferably when everyone is happy and relaxed. For most families, this is morning time when the baby is happy and when the mother has the highest level of "mother" hormones.
- Practice for 10-15 minutes with your baby, doing your best to keep everyone happy.
- If your baby becomes sad, do not breastfeed right away. Instead, comfort and distract your baby, then breastfeed about 10 minutes later, so your baby does not associate refusing the bottle with winning the breast.
- When your baby *does* accept the bottle and will eat about 2 ounces, it is okay to finish the feeding with breastfeeding.
- If you have already found the best bottle nipple "fit" as suggested in Chapter 6, it is not necessary to purchase more bottle nipple varieties. Consistency in offering the nipple you have is a better choice.

Give each idea you try two or three feedings to work before trying another idea.

Position

- If your baby will accept the bottle from mom, but not from dad, try handing the baby off during a feeding and offering the bottle "together."
- Try different feeding positions in your arms: baby's back leaning on adult's chest, baby "sitting" on adult's lap, baby facing adult.
- Try different feeding positions while *not* being held: in the baby swing, in a bouncy chair, on the couch, in a stroller, in the car seat.

Location

- Feed outside while looking at the trees, bushes, or clouds (try both in your arms and out of your arms).
- Choose a place to bottle-feed where your baby does not breastfeed (not the rocker or nursing "corner").
- Introduce the bottle while your baby is in the bath.

Timing

- Offer the bottle about 30 minutes after breastfeeding, when your baby is awake, but not hungry.
- Offer the bottle when your baby shows signs of being hungry.
- Offer the bottle when your baby awakens from a nap, still slightly groggy and wanting to breastfeed.
- Offer the bottle for a middle-of-the-night feeding using the above strategies: either start with a bottle at the beginning of a feeding, switching to breastfeeding after baby eats an ounce, or start with breastfeeding and after the first let-down at the breast, finish the feeding with the bottle.

Associations & Distractions

- Sing the same song at feeding time: sing to your baby before you feed, and sing once more while you feed. Singing while you breastfeed may help your baby associate this song with feeding from the bottle. This association can transfer between mom, dad, and caregiver.
- Hide the bottle with a small blanket, washcloth, or stuffed animal. When you find a cover you and your baby prefer, continue to use the same bottle "cover" for association. Consider buying a stack of washcloths (the same color) to send with your baby to daycare for consistency, and to double as a burp cloth (hence, more than one).
- Swaddle your baby in a blanket or piece of clothing (nightshirt) that smells like mom.

Nipple Switch

- While your baby nurses to sleep, remove your nipple from the baby's mouth and replace it with the bottle nipple.
- While your baby is nursing during a wakeful time of day, try replacing your nipple with the bottle *after* the first let-down, so your baby's initial hunger is satisfied with breastfeeding.
- If your baby uses a pacifier, try replacing the pacifier with the bottle nipple.
- If your baby is willing to suck on your finger, slip the bottle in while the baby is sucking. This will affect the mouth placement temporarily, but might get the baby over the hump.

Other Points to Consider

- If your baby is older than 3-4 months, be sure he is willing to accept things other than the breast in his mouth: teether toys, blankies, stuffed animals, washcloths, etc.

Do Not

- *Do not* engage in bottle battles that involve a screaming baby and a frustrated daddy—your baby needs to associate his dad with happy activities. If interaction with dad is saved for learning to bottle-feed, your baby might think his daddy is the cause of sadness.
- *Do not* let the baby get "good and hungry" so he takes the bottle—this is a very harsh idea. There are numerous *kind* ways to encourage your baby to take a bottle, rather than starving him.
- *Do not* replace breastmilk with formula or juice thinking perhaps the baby does not want to taste breastmilk from a different source. This is not a good idea because this jeopardizes the lining of your baby's intestines, sets your baby up for tummy woes, and exposes your baby to early allergens.
- *Do not* let the caregiver figure out how to feed your baby—leaving your baby can feel worrisome in itself; adding the layer of, "Will my baby eat?" creates more stress.
- *Do not* plan to feed your baby long-term with a syringe, eye-dropper, or medicine cup—babies like and need to suck. If you will be away from your baby for several feedings in a row, finding a bottle baby will take can make everyone happier: baby, caregiver, and parents.
- *Do not* switch to a higher flow nipple—pouring milk into your baby's mouth is essentially force feeding, creating an unhappy experience and a risk for aspiration and choking.

Glossary

Abrupt widening: a marked transition from the nipple tip to the nipple base, preventing the baby's lips from resting on a portion of the nipple base

All-or-none: choosing to stop breastfeeding if a baby drinks some formula; based on the misconception that the benefits of breastmilk are lost once a baby is given formula

Areola: the pinkish-brown skin surrounding the nipple

Artificial nipple: a non-human nipple; bottle nipple or pacifier

Assess: to observe, evaluate, judge, and make changes accordingly

Baby-led feeding: a feeding style that is guided by the baby's movements and instinctive feeding behaviors

Beveled-shape nipple: rounded on one side with a flat, diagonal slope on the other; resembling a tube of lipstick

Bottle strike: when a baby who formerly would eat from a bottle suddenly refuses

Bottle system: using the same brand of bottle nipple, collar, and bottle; also called feeding system

Breastmilk substitute: formula; artificial baby milk

Breastfeeding goals: how long a mother plans to breastfeed her baby and/or pump her breastmilk

Breastfeeding meal: a full feeding at the breast

Butterfly shape: flat and wide pacifier nipple

Cherry shape: pacifier shape with a bulbous tip and narrowed base

Collar: the ring that a bottle nipple fits into, which then screws onto the bottle

Colostrum: first milk, present in the breast at the end of pregnancy and when the baby is born

Compress: change the shape of an object by applying pressure and/or squeezing

Cycles: number of times per minute a breast pump sucks and releases

Ducts: channels that carry milk from the breast to the nipple; also see plugged duct

Engorgement: overly full breasts that may feel warm, hard, and uncomfortable; the fullness or swelling results from milk that has not been removed, as well as increased blood flow

Equalization: to make equal in pressure; evidenced with a bottle if it stops dripping after five seconds of inverting

Express: to remove milk from the breast with a breast pump or with the mother's hand (manually)

Feeding cues: ways a baby communicates hunger, such as smacking or licking lips, putting a fist near the mouth, rooting on a blanket, or episodes of light sleep

Feeding method: process by which a baby is fed; breast, bottle, or a combination

Feeding system: using the same brand of bottle nipple, collar, and bottle; also called bottle system

Filter: the small piece of the breast pump that attaches between the flange and bottle which milk drips through; sometimes called a membrane

Flange, breast pump: the part of the breast pump that is held to your breast as you pump

Flange, lips: top and bottom lips roll outward like a fish, sealing on the breast or bottle

Flow: the rate milk comes out of the breast or bottle; bottle companies also call this size or flow-rate

Flow preference: when a baby favors one feeding method over another due to how fast the milk is delivered

Formula feedings: using formula rather than breastmilk to feed a baby

Gradual widening: a gentle transition from the nipple tip to the nipple base, allowing for correct mouth placement

Growth spurt: when a baby feeds frequently at the breast, usually for 2 or 3 days, to increase his mother's milk supply

Hindmilk: the milk excreted by the breast during the last portion of a feeding or pumping session; higher in fat than foremilk

Interactive feeding: applying some elements of baby-led feeding to mother-led feeding, bringing a balance to the mother-led style, so a baby's instinctive feeding behaviors are not ignored

Inverting: angling a bottle down to allow it to equalize in pressure and stop dripping

Latching: when a baby is grasping the nipple and areola for feeding and/or sucking

Let-down: when the milk ejection reflex occurs as the cells within the breast contract and eject milk

Membrane: the small piece of the breast pump, attaching between the flange and bottle, which milk drips through; sometimes called a filter

Milk-ejection reflex: also called let-down, when the cells within the breast contract and eject milk

Mother-led feeding: a feeding style that is guided by the mother's movements; how she positions her baby, supports her breast, and quickly helps her baby latch

Mouth placement: where the nipple rests in the baby's mouth, and how the baby's lips and tongue accept the nipple

Narrow neck: also called standard; bottle nipples that have a smaller base; many narrow neck nipples and bottles are interchangeable

Nipple: (human) the center, cylindrical portion of the breast, from which the milk flows

Nipple base: the lower portion of an artificial nipple meant to mimic a human areola; the baby's lips are intended to rest gently on a portion of the nipple base

Nipple confusion: when a baby can't remember to change his suck from one type of nipple to another; often caused by poor nipple selection and feeding techniques that do not support breastfeeding

Nipple length: the cylindrical part of an artificial nipple that is in contact with the baby's tongue

Nipple preference: when a baby prefers the texture, shape, or flow of one nipple over another

Nipple tip: the end of an artificial nipple where the milk flows out

No-drip: an artificial nipple that does not leak milk when the bottle is tipped down; many artificial nipples equalize and become no-drip nipples after five seconds of inversion

Non-nutritive sucking: rapid, short sucks when a baby begins breastfeeding, sometimes called flutter sucking; provides stimulation of the nipples which causes a let-down

Nursing strike: when a breastfeeding baby suddenly refuses to breastfeed

Nutritive sucking: slow, long sucks usually with audible swallowing; follows non-nutritive sucking

Orthodontic: a shape of bottle nipple or pacifier that is rounded on one side with a flat, diagonal slope on the other; resembling a tube of lipstick

Palate: the roof of a baby's mouth; the hard palate is in the front portion of the mouth behind the upper gum ridge, while the soft palate is the arch in the back portion of the mouth

Plugged duct: an area of the breast where milk flow is obstructed, resulting in a tender lump beneath the tissue

Postpartum depression: a medical diagnosis that includes baby blues, depression, or psychosis of a mother within the first year following childbirth

Pumping: using a machine to express breastmilk

Retracted: when a baby's tongue tip is pulled behind the lower gum ridge, and mid-tongue reaches toward the soft palate; often causes a biting reflex

Rooting: when a baby opens his mouth and searches for a nipple to grasp; this is a reflex the baby is born with

Shallow placement: when a baby holds a nipple in the front of his mouth; poor placement

SIMPLE Method: an acronym identifying the various steps in choosing the best bottle nipple for a breastfed baby according to the baby's unique suck characteristics

Simulating let-downs: mimicking let-downs that occur naturally at the breast with a bottle to support breastfeeding and reduce nipple preference

Snack-time: offering a small-quantity with a bottle between typical breastfeeding times

Stockpiling: combining the milk from two or more pumping sessions; or to build a surplus of frozen milk in the freezer for later use

Supplement: additional milk fed to a baby, breastmilk or formula

Supply and demand: the amount of breastmilk a mother produces determined in part by how much milk is removed from the breast

Texture: how a nipple feels, ranging from soft and squishy to stiff

Tongue cupping: the cradling action of a baby's tongue around a nipple length

Vacuum: the suction action of a breast pump

Vent: allows the air pressure to equalize in a bottle as a baby sucks

Weaning: the process of gradually stopping breastfeeding, bottle-feeding, or pacifier use

Wide neck: bottle nipples that have a wide base and work with fatter bottles

Index

I

L

M

N

O

P

R

S

T

V

W

Author Bios

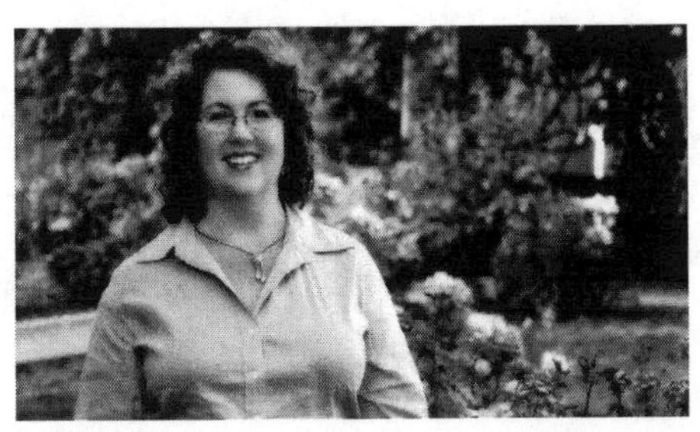

Amy Peterson is an IBCLC in private practice. She has worked with breastfeeding mothers since 1996, professionally since 2001. Her practice primarily consists of difficult breastfeeding cases, including disorganized and dysfunctional sucks. Amy enjoys being an advocate for mothers who need encouragement to help them reach their breastfeeding goals. She often works side-by-side with co-author Mindy, a Speech-Language Pathologist, bringing a wider scope of service to her mother-baby clients. In addition to co-authoring *Balancing Breast and Bottle: Reaching Your Breastfeeding Goals*, she is co-author of "Taking Care of Your Breastfed Babies' Teeth," published in the *Journal of Human Lactation (2008),* and enjoys speaking at lactation conferences. Amy earned her Bachelor of Science degree in Education from the University of Texas in Austin. She lives in Jerome, Idaho, with her husband and their four children.

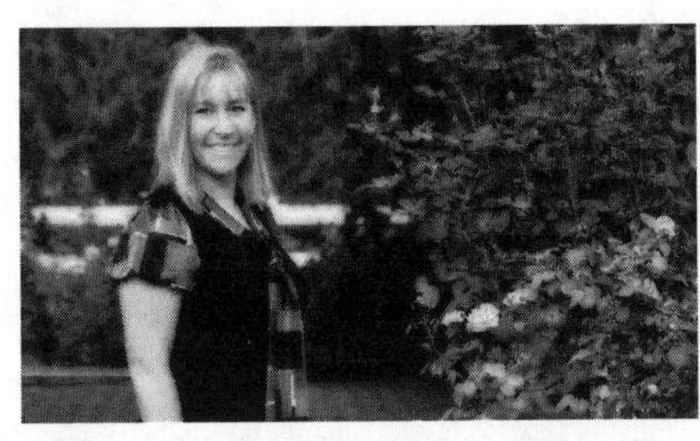

Mindy Harmer received her Master of Arts in Speech and Hearing Sciences from the University of California, Santa Barbara, and went on to do additional graduate work at Vanderbilt University in the early 1990s. She has practiced in the field of speech-language pathology for the past 15 years as a private practitioner, specializing in pediatrics. Mindy is co-owner of Cierra Therapy where she treats clients with a variety of speech-language and feeding disorders. Some of her tiniest clients are breastfeeding babies who require her knowledge of oral-motor intervention to help them breastfeed successfully. She became interested in breastfeeding when she was encouraged to pump breastmilk for her son who was born with a congenital heart defect. Mindy resides in Twin Falls, Idaho, with her husband, Eric Herzog, and their two children.

Pictures by Clark Draney

Ordering Information

Hale Publishing, L.P.
1825 E Plano Parkway, Suite 280
Plano, Texas 75074

8:00 AM to 5:00 PM CST

Call » 972.578.0400
Fax » 972.578.0413

Online
www.HalePublishing.com